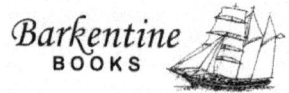

The Road to Kidneyville

A Journey through Diabetes, Dialysis, and Transplant

By Jesse Crain

About the Author

Jesse Crain was never trained as a nurse, and in fact, had no desire to be one. But circumstances and the health needs of her husband forced a need for knowledge and a skill set that had nothing to do with her desires.

Jesse loves animals, reading, living the country life, and especially her family, near and far. She has always lived in Missouri.

TABLE OF CONTENTS

INTRODUCTION

In April 2008 my husband Larry began dialysis treatments for End-Stage Renal Disease (ESRD). It's a terrifying name, isn't it? Those first two words... well, let's hope that someday, with advances in modern medicine, the term will become obsolete. But as of now it is not, and therefore, this memoir.

When Larry started dialysis and the idea of him "someday" undergoing a kidney transplant gradually became more than a nebulous concept to us, I began looking for books that might tell us what to expect. I found one book by a physician who had also become a dialysis and subsequent transplant patient, and another by a Hollywood VIP; neither book seemed appropriate to our level of knowledge or privilege.

Finally, in the summer of 2011, while setting up the machine for the almost-nightly ritual of dialysis, I told Larry we should write a book. A book about what it's like for the patient who is on dialysis, and also what it's like for the parent, spouse, or sibling who assists with dialysis, as well as with the doctor and nurse visits, the frequent calls and emails, and the entire transplant process: trying to get on the transplant list for a kidney, then staying on the list, and last (hopefully!) to someday actually getting a working kidney. I told Larry that maybe we could help other people who were (or soon would be) going through this situation. I even popped off with a potential title.

Larry looked up at me through his long eyelashes with a straight face.

"Well, you could write a book." He didn't need to remind me that he rarely read a book, let alone that he'd never aspire to write one. Of his many strong points, literature was not among them.

"OK, so I will write the book, and read the parts to you as it's written so you can add or correct or whatever, and it will be a team effort" I told him.

"Hmm. Whatever you think."

So here it is. It is my sincere hope that this will be useful and encouraging to those who are now walking down a path that is sometimes dark and often fraught with worry and uncertainty. In some small way I hope it imparts knowledge they may not have had access to otherwise. For me it has become an outlet for my own remembrances and I hope a tribute to Larry.

My most humble thanks to all who assisted with the details. A few names have been changed in some anecdotes. Any errors in particulars are my own, for which I beg pardon. This is one man's story, or at least a part of it. An imperfect human like the rest of us, but a man with a generous heart, a warrior spirit, a protective nature, and an eye for the beauty of life and the wonder of God's creation. Larry, my beau, this is for you.

1
THE EARLY YEARS

Maybe she was the prettiest thing he'd ever seen.

Burl Crain's first glimpse of Nadine Bonewell was at a little country rodeo on a ranch in southeast Colorado. He was on someone else's horse and she wanted a ride, so he helped her up into the saddle and sat behind her. They rode, talked, laughed—had a good time.

He didn't see her again until the next summer, at another rodeo. She remembered him and it was clear the mutual attraction was still there, so he asked her out on a date. They were both of pioneer stock, and shared similar backgrounds. Both had grown up with farm chores: "Feed the horses, gather the eggs, milk the cows, and check the fences. And watch out for rattlesnakes!"—because this is dry, rocky country, almost to New Mexico.

The War Years were just past. Electricity was making its way to the rural areas—the teenaged Burl helped his daddy put up poles. Ranching was hard work, but he looked forward to those Saturday evening dates with Nadine. They were a couple for a few months. He proposed; she said yes. There followed, in rapid order, a November wedding in 1948, a brief honeymoon trip to California, and a 10-pound baby boy born October 5, 1949. Burl named him Larry Dean.

There was no way they could know, as they gazed with wonder on this brand new miracle they'd created, where his future would lead him.

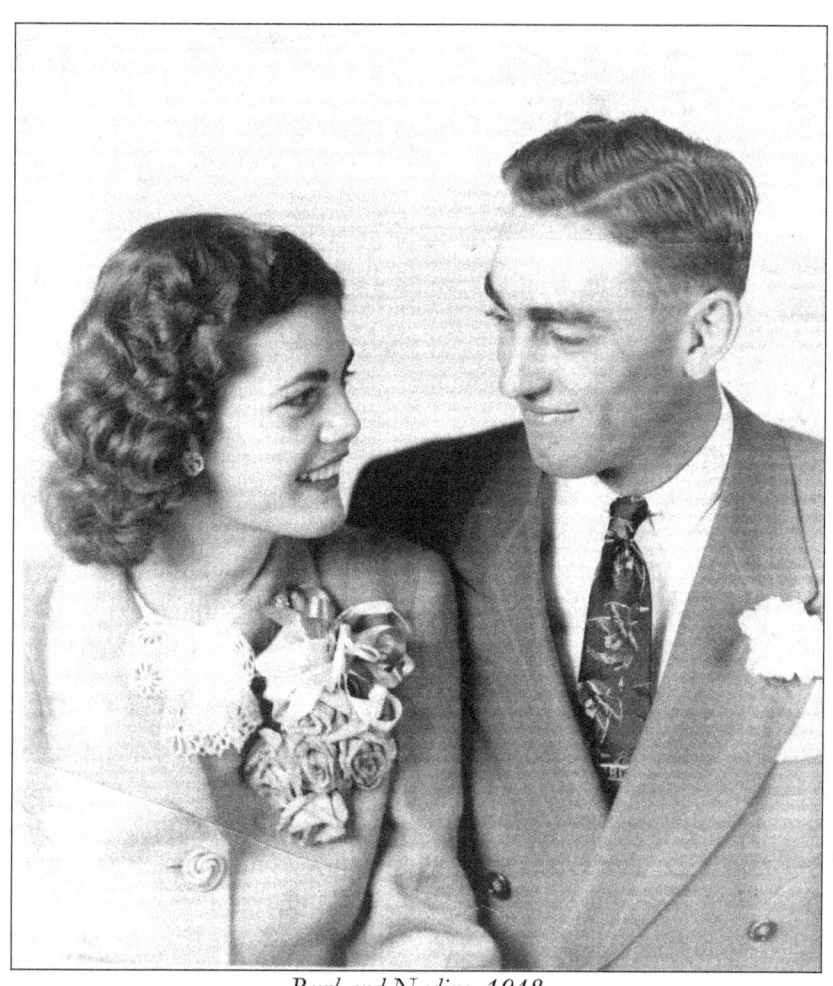

Burl and Nadine, 1948

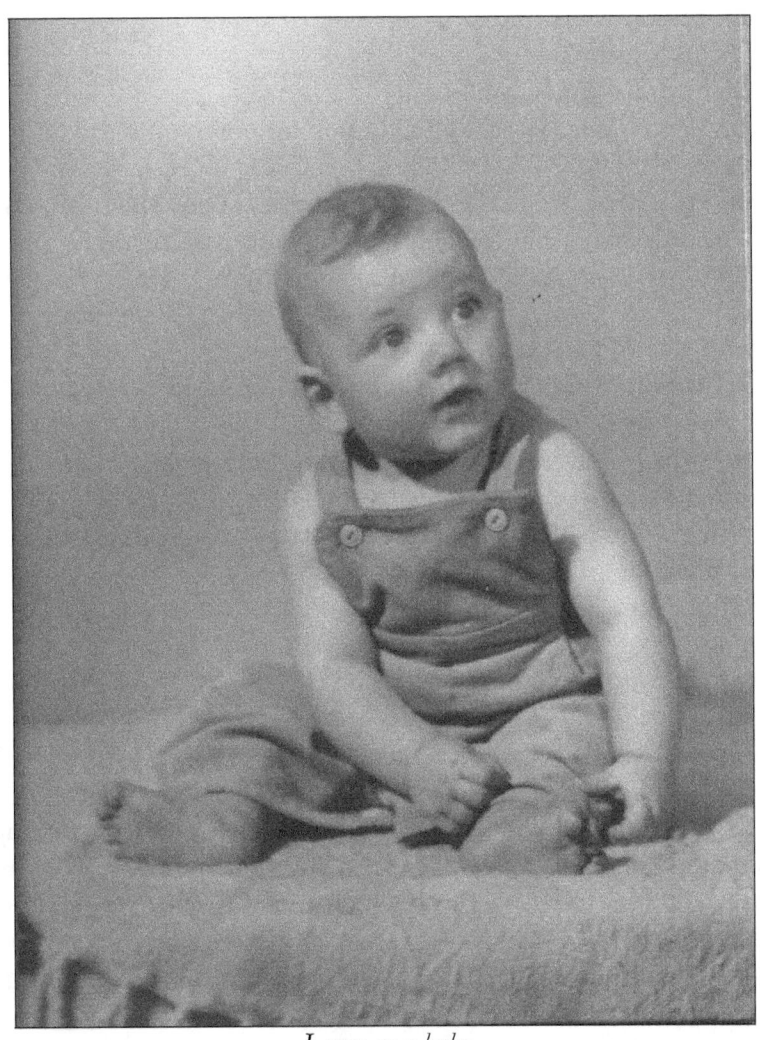

Larry as a baby

* * *

Sometimes children are born with obvious health problems. Sometimes illness shows its face with slow symptoms that are difficult to diagnose, or even see. But in Larry's case it was a sudden wake-up call—or, rather, an attempted wake-up—that told them something was definitely wrong. Larry was 5 years old in the fall of 1954, his brother Tommy was almost 3, and sister Susan was 1. Nadine went to see why Larry wasn't up yet, and she couldn't rouse him.

Yes, he was breathing.

No, he didn't feel feverish.

She was sure he wasn't playing possum. Why in the world was he not responding?!

Nadine called the family doctor they'd found when the family had moved that year to Colorado Springs, after trading some furniture for a down payment on a mobile home. This was back in the day when family doctors still made house calls, and so the doctor drove right over.

"I don't know what's wrong with him", the doctor told her, "but I know someone who will."

Burl was called home from work, and they bundled Larry up in blankets and drove him to Penrose Hospital. It didn't take the pediatrician long to diagnose the problem: "sugar diabetes," also called juvenile or Type 1 diabetes.

Insulin was administered, but at this point it was anybody's guess how much would do the job on Larry's little body. It took almost 3 days of cautious dosing before the boy woke up in the middle of the night, and *gee whiz,* was he *HUNGRY!*

Some of the nurses were nuns, and Larry often recalled his "guardian angel" that night as young, pretty, and sweet natured, wearing the long white habit and wimple of her order. She brought him a single-serving box of cereal with a half-pint carton of milk and a spoon. The snack was consumed rapidly, with more requested. She complied, only to hear the same question: "More?" This time she had to hurry across the street to an all-night quick shop, returning with a full-sized box of cereal and half a gallon of milk.

Larry finished both.

* * *

10

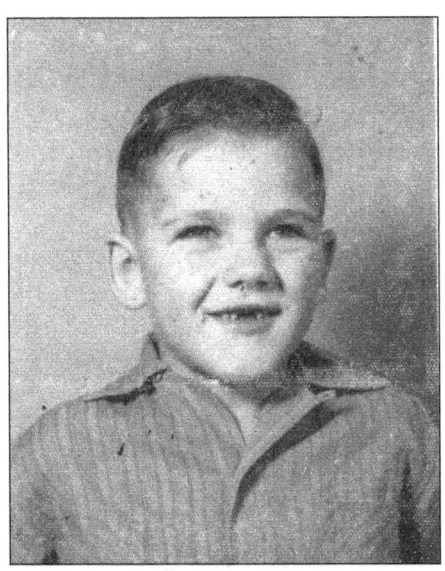

Larry, age 7

Prior to the 1920s a diagnosis of diabetes mellitus was a death sentence. Most children who were found to have this disease before the age of seven were given a prognosis of two more years to live, at the most, with younger patients frequently succumbing sooner. The discovery in 1921 of insulin injections as a treatment for diabetes was considered a true miracle by many patients and their families. At first insulin was obtained from animals (cows, horses, pigs, even fish), and problems with refining and purification had to be worked out. Still—can you imagine the excitement of their doctors, too, to be able to offer this hope?

Before taking Larry home, Burl and Nadine had to learn how to draw up and give Larry's insulin shots. He was given one shot of insulin each morning. The syringes were glass, the needles stainless steel, and both had to be sterilized by boiling in water for 20 minutes after each use. The needles were large and long, and from time to time Burl had to sharpen them on a whetstone. Single-use syringes were not introduced until 1961, and not readily available—or affordable—in all areas right away. Because the handheld glucose monitors so easily obtained today hadn't even been invented yet, there were lots of trips back to the hospital as they tried to regulate Larry's glucose levels. Like most kids he enjoyed sweets, and didn't understand why he wasn't supposed to have them. Burl says sometimes they gave in to their son's pleas to be allowed to share in a birthday cake or Christmas cookies, but then administered an extra shot of the insulin to make up for it. Once, unknown to his parents, Larry got hold of a bag of Red Hots, his favorite cinnamon candy, and polished off the entire contents. He knew his mama would be mad... and he was right. Nadine wanted to tan his hide when she found out.

The summer Larry was 7, he wanted to go for an extended visit with his maternal grandparents. Grandma and Granddad had a farm, with room to run and play and a pond for fishing. Grandma thought she could use his help in the garden, but this no-nonsense woman who could build herself a cabinet if she wanted one was squeamish about having to stab her eldest grandchild with needles every day. Nadine showed Larry how the process worked. Grandma would sterilize the syringes, but Larry would have to give himself the insulin shots.

It was his responsibility from then on.

* * *

Larry's first school fight came when he was in the fifth grade. He was a minority student at the grade school he attended, and a 6th grade boy approached him one day, accused Larry of "messing with" the older boy's sister, and beat him up. Two things made Larry mad; the obvious embarrassment of being caught unprepared to defend himself, and the injustice of being wrongfully blamed for something he'd not done. Heck, he hadn't even *wanted* to!

After the thrashing, as he walked down the hall toward the double doors to leave, Larry's anger boiled over. He doubled up his 10-year-old fist and punched the door of the school restroom, breaking a hole in the hollow-core wood. A teacher saw it, the principal was consulted, and Dad was called. Larry told him what had happened.

"Well son," Burl said, "if you'd hit the bigger kid the way you hit that door, he'd have probably left you alone!"

That evening at home they worked on defense.

Larry delivered papers to pay for the door.

In the days that followed, as Larry progressed in his lessons in defense, Burl showed him how to block punches from an attacker and how to hit back. "Then don't quit hitting back 'till he's on the ground." He showed him where to hit (shoulders, stomach, face), and how to hit so as to minimize injury to himself.

"If you hit with your knuckles very often, it'll hurt like hell," his dad told him. "Instead, use the heel of your palm or your forearm, down close to, but not right on, your elbow. Try to get up under his nose, or chin."

Burl also told him not to start fights, but not to be afraid to settle them either. As the eldest son, Larry was also charged with the typical duty of watching after the younger siblings. Tom, Susan, and other kids at school and in the neighborhood quickly learned to call on Larry's assistance when confronted with a bully.

He never let them down.

*   *   *

Grade school flew by, then the junior high years. One summer Robbie, the oldest boy in the neighborhood, was teaching the younger kids how to do the "Western Roll", a high-jump maneuver in which an athlete runs at an angle toward a horizontal pole (such as a high jumper would use), dives over it hands first, then tucks his arms, lands on his inward-curled shoulder, and rolls into the sand pit beyond. These would-be athletes, however, were in the vacant lot behind their yards. Eight or 10 boys were in the group and had dug up the hard-packed dirt for the pit, but it was probably only 1 to 2 inches deep; "we thought we were tough," Larry said. They'd rigged the pole stand with a couple of forked tree branches for the uprights; the horizontal bar was a bamboo pole on which a roll of carpet had been delivered. Larry lined up for his turn, ran as fast as he could, and propelled himself into the jump. Airborne! He was over the bar, clearing it easily. Then the goof: he forgot to tuck his arms. When he landed hard on the left forearm, every boy on the lot heard the *snap!* of the bone breaking.

The rest of that summer Larry's arm was in a cast. So much for sports that vacation.

13

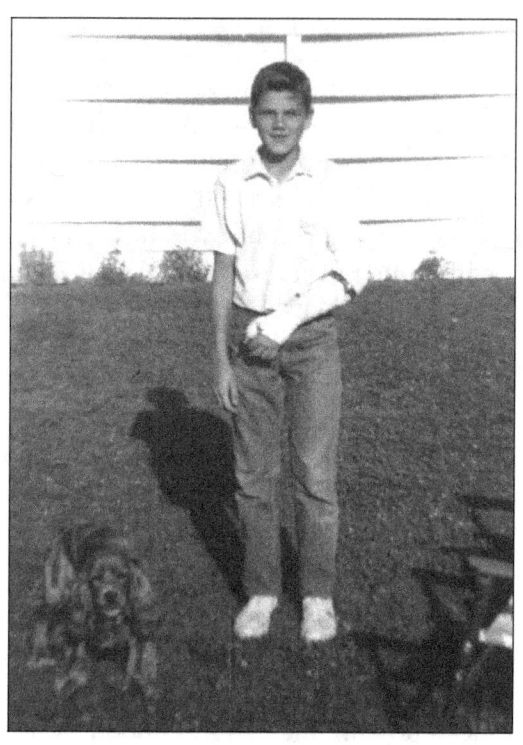

Unhappy Landing

* * *

Then one morning when Larry was 13 or so, Nadine went to wake him up and found him once again in an insulin reaction—not unconscious, but woozy and uncooperative. Not having enough glucose ("sugar") in the bloodstream can often cause an inability to concentrate or think clearly because brain cells do not store excess glucose and need a continual supply. Burl mixed some sugar into a glass of water. He slid his arm under the pillow and supported Larry's head while Nadine raised the glass to their son's lips and implored him to drink. What happened next shocked them both: Larry bit a chunk out of the rim of the glass and began chewing it up! Burl tried to get a finger in to sweep the glass fragments out of Larry's mouth, but the boy's sugar-deprived brain had him fighting back, shaking his head from side to side, flailing out with his arms, twisting his body away from what must have seemed like an attack. All he wanted to do was slip back into the oblivion of sleep, and here were these people, shouting at him!

So they made another trip to the hospital. Glucose was administered to bring Larry around. Burl thought surely the boy's stomach should be pumped, but the doctors said no, that he'd be alright.

After that, only plastic or metal tumblers were used to give Larry liquids when he was "low." It's a precaution our entire family observed thereafter... always.

* * *

By the time he was in his mid-teens, Larry was lank and tall, with big hands and long feet. Many of the men in his dad's family were tall, lean, and sinewy, reminiscent of their ancestors who'd migrated from South Carolina after the Revolutionary War, moving east to Tennessee and Texas, then homesteading in Colorado as Burl's dad had. They were a hardworking bunch for whom weakness was almost akin to laziness, which would've been inexcusable. If you wanted something, you worked for it. Well, Larry wanted to look like those muscle men he'd seen on TV. Now, how to work for that?

The physical education teacher at his high school offered the use of the weight-lifting equipment, so Larry and younger brother Tom began staying after classes, working out and building muscle. Coach said they could really pack on the pounds by eating a can of pork 'n' beans every day, so they did. Larry worked hard to develop that "V" shape to his back, wide at the shoulders and narrow at the hips. His arms weren't as big as he wanted them to be, but they were getting strong. A pair of older boys, brothers Jim and Robbie, could press 200 pounds each, and they taught Larry what to do. Pretty soon he could bench press more than 200 pounds as well.

* * *

The summer Larry was almost 15, Burl's friend Jim was putting together a crew for wheat harvest. He had the combines and the grain trucks, a flatbed semi to haul equipment, an old school bus

15

he'd converted to a rolling bunkhouse, and a travel trailer for himself and his wife, who cooked all the meals for the crew. Jim had contracted work from farmers all the way from Oklahoma to North Dakota, and agreed to put Larry on his crew. It was his first full-time summer job. They started on wheat fields in the Panhandle and worked their way north as the season progressed. On rainy days they sat in the bus and played cards, but mostly they worked long hours to get the crop harvested. Larry arrived back at home tanned, confident, and stronger than ever.

During this time Larry and Tom would visit the arcade in Manitou Springs to play skeeball, pinball, and pool. They especially relished the challenge of the arm wrestling machine. After Larry's grip and strength broke three of the units in 3 months, the arcade banned them from that particular pleasure.

* * *

Although Larry and Tom both inherited their dad's raw-boned sinewy height, sister Susan echoed Nadine's petite build. At 5'1" and slender, Susan was bright-eyed, fresh-faced, and cute. But one of the guys who asked her out was not so cute. He was taller than Larry. He was heavy. He was a bully and so was his best friend, who was known to be a tough guy around school. The fact that Susan told him "no" didn't mean much to Fred. He said "Oh, you're gonna go out with me alright. Be ready at 7 o'clock." And he walked off.

At 7:00 o'clock Fred came to the house, backed up by his friends. Susan had told Larry all about it, so he knew she had no desire to go out with this pushy so-and-so. When the car pulled up in the street out front, Larry instructed Susan to stay in the house, and then he went out onto the sidewalk. Tom stepped out behind his big brother, knowing Larry probably didn't need any help, but showing his solidarity anyway.

Larry was clear. "She's not going out with you. Get back in your car and leave."

"No." Fred said, "I came to pick up Susan, and I'm not leaving without her."

"Susan is not going anywhere with you." Big brother had

spoken.

Fred poked two fingers into Larry's chest. "She's gonna get in my car."

"No, she's not gonna get in your car, your pal's car, or anybody else's car if she doesn't want to," Larry said, and gave Fred's chest a poke in return. His blue eyes were intense and showed no fear. "You should leave. Now."

One of Fred's back-ups finally said "Come on, Fred, there's no point arguing about this; let's go. You don't want to get into it with this guy. He's not afraid of you and he'll knock you on your ass."

They left. Susan wasn't bothered again.

* * *

At that time, kids in Colorado could get a motorcycle license at 14, and Larry hadn't hesitated. The first time he really noticed motorcycles, he was 5 years old and the family was visiting his paternal grandmother, Kate. Her back yard had a chain link fence, and beyond the fence was some open land and a highway. Larry and Tom were playing in the backyard when they heard—and felt—an approaching rumble coming up the road. They ran to the fence, latching on with their little fingers and the toes of their sneakers to climb higher and see better as a group of two or three dozen motorcycles came into view. Wow! The fence they clung to seemed to shake with the vibration of all those loud engines. Like as not the bikers didn't notice a pair of little boys; but the boys sure were taking in the bikes... and for Larry, it was love.

So, it was no surprise to Burl when Larry announced at 14 that he had saved up some money and was going to buy a bike—and not the bicycle kind.

* * *

To a lot of folks, motorcycles are a symbol of freedom, as close as they feel they can come to soaring like an eagle. Larry loved birds, had raised pigeons as a boy and loved to watch hawks, eagles, geese, anything moving through the sky. How would it feel to be up there, gliding and soaring? Well, his motorcycle gave him a taste of that, even if it was on the highway. But being young and free and flying down the highway on your motorcycle can be more than freedom: It can be trouble.

Tom was riding on the Honda 450, perched behind Larry. They were with a friend, Roger, who had his own bike, and had stopped outside Pueblo at a fast food joint to take a break when they saw a second friend, Robert—RC, they called him—ride by in the direction of Colorado Springs. The three of them hurried to jump back on their bikes to catch up to him. It was a divided highway with a grassy median between the east- and westbound lanes, and a 70-mph speed limit. But hey, the bikes would do 85, maybe 90! Now they were really on the wing.

Until the state trooper caught sight of them from the opposite side of the highway.

The flashing lights came on, the cruiser made a left turn across the grass, and on it came, siren wailing.

"Larry, you gotta stop!" Tom leaned up and spoke urgently into his big brother's ear.

"But Roger's up ahead over that hill; he won't know what happened to us," Larry argued.

"Well, maybe *he* can get outta this, but *we* can't" Tom said.

They slowed to pull over, but the trooper didn't. He pulled up right next to them, motioned for them to pull over and stay put, and went after their companion up ahead. The boys just stared at the cruiser as it sped out again, in hot pursuit of Roger.

"Tom?" Larry hesitated but a second, "maybe we *can* get out of this."

Larry watched the trooper disappear over the hill, then stomped on the brake, checked behind him for traffic, and made his own left turn across the grassy strip and into the eastbound lane, twisting the throttle for quick speed. He went a short distance to a rest area where there was a slight incline off to the side of the road; there Larry carefully maneuvered the bike up the rise of weeds and rock, over the knoll, and out of sight of the highway. They got down on their bellies behind some brush where they could watch the traffic without being seen, like Indians on watch for the cavalry.

"Dad's gonna have our hides for this," Tom groaned.

"Maybe so, but at least the cops won't have my license," Larry replied.

They waited. They watched. There he was. The trooper was heading east again, with Roger right behind him. It looked like they were going to the local office in Pueblo. Larry and Tom hid out until dark.

"Come on, let's go," Larry said, and they eased the motorcycle back down the hill and across the median, watching over their shoulders just in case. Then they were on the road again, and made it to LaJunta, to RC's house. Somehow they found a sympathetic ear in RC's dad. They spent the night there, and he fixed the boys breakfast in the morning. He helped them load the Honda into the bed of his pickup, then covered it with a tarp and drove the boys back to Colorado Springs and home. Burl broke the news that a trooper had already been there looking for them, thanks to information apparently given up by Roger. *Couldn't he just have pretended he was alone and didn't know who was riding behind him?* they wondered.

"You boys better lay low and sing small for a while." Burl told them. "Leave that motorcycle in the garage. Sounds like it'll be a hot target for a few days at least."

* * *

Having his own wheels also meant Larry could ride up into the mountains to climb the rocks and hike the trails. His love of nature had been encouraged with camping, fishing and hunting trips with his parents from the time he was young. The problem came when he cut classes at school in order to indulge these hobbies.

"If you don't graduate high school, you won't amount to much," he was told.

But he wasn't particularly studious. He didn't enjoy reading. He didn't intend to go to college. Didn't want to enter the corporate job force. Couldn't see that a high school diploma was going to make a big difference in his life.

Like many teenagers, Larry rebelled. And just like many kids in the 1960s, he started growing his hair long. Typical of most dads of the era, Burl didn't like it and it became one of their running arguments.

The family was having other issues, too, that affected Larry. All marriages go through rough spots, and Larry's parents' marriage was no different. The rough spots, however, had turned into major problems, and the pair separated, then divorced. The kids stayed in the house with Burl. Nadine moved to Canon City, where she had family. Previously she had often tried to run interference between her husband and her eldest son, but now she wasn't there to break up the fights.

Smoking also became part of Larry's life. Both Burl and Nadine smoked cigarettes then; in the mid-1960s, almost half of American adults did. Larry started out by liberating a few from his mom's pack here and there, but by 16 he was smoking openly and regularly. Did the doctors at that time know how harmful this could be, and how much riskier this was for a person with Type 1 diabetes? If so, did Larry see a doctor who told him these things? And if so, did he listen? Probably not, at least to the last of those questions. A typical 16-year-old is invincible, right?

The arguments at home escalated. Burl had a grown-up's perspective and Larry had a teenager's defiance. The result wasn't easy on either of them.

Larry found an apartment in an old house across town that had been converted to several small units. It was far from luxury, but he finally felt he could make his own rules. He stayed in high school, but was not what you might call scholarly. He worked after-school and weekend jobs wherever he could find employment: in the laundry at the Union Printers' Home, cleaning up the restaurant at the airport, walking a pair of St. Bernard dogs for a guy who worked nights.

And he graduated.

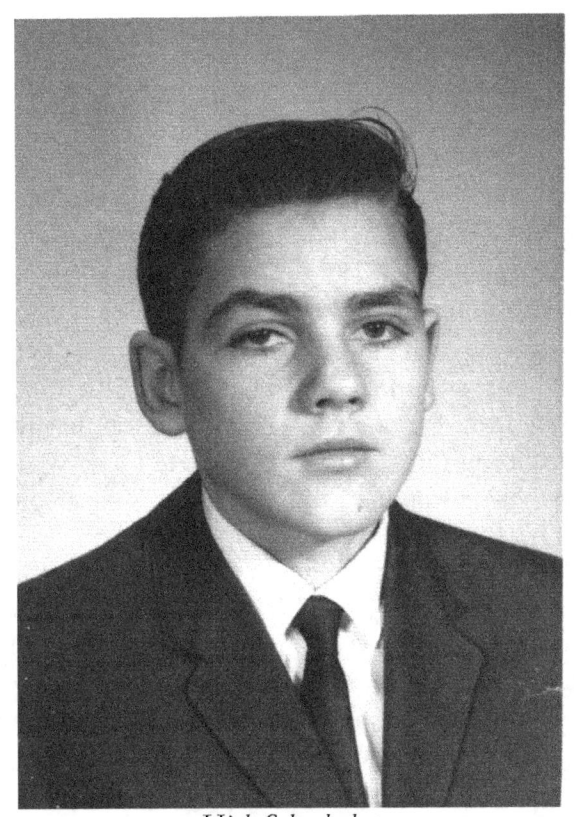

High School photo

2
TAP-BOOM!

Remember those little wooden toys they used to sell that looked like miniature workbenches and had a tiny wooden mallet along with several wooden pegs of various shapes? The idea was to match the pegs to coordinating holes and then tap them with the mallet to get the peg through the hole and into the box below. Maybe they even fell into the category of educational toys for toddlers because matching the pegs to the holes would foster deductive reasoning, and hammering them through the holes would promote hand-eye coordination and motor skills. OK, so maybe that's reaching a bit. But anyway, Larry told me that when he was little he went through three of those sets. He *loved* whacking away at those pegs. And bless his folks for buying the second and third ones after he beat the first two to a pulp!

After wheat harvest and weightlifting and odd jobs around here and there, Larry somehow found his way into the carpentry field. When the North American Air Defense Command (NORAD) was being built inside Cheyenne Mountain, he and Tom got jobs carrying sheetrock (or drywall, as it is also called) in to the job site. They would compete to see who could carry the most at a time. But what attracted Larry's attention most were the framers; the good ones could really drive those nails fast, straight, and accurate—no nail guns in those days.

Before long Larry had a job with a building crew, putting up houses and apartment buildings. He learned to drive a 16-penny nail into a pair of 2×4s with a light starter hit to set it, then a massive blow to sink it in up to the head: tap-BOOM, then move on to the next: tap-BOOM. He was good, and he enjoyed it. Seeing the daily progress of a building going up as a result of labor he put in with the other guys made him proud. It was hard work, but that never bothered him. Just give him a good stout hammer and a tool belt with nails in the pouch and turn him loose. tap-BOOM!

The winds whistling down off the mountains around Colorado

Springs could be a challenge, though. One day he and his boss had finished the framing on a two-story house and were nailing the plywood decking on the roof. Larry picked up a 4x8 sheet of plywood, balanced it on his head with one hand gripping each long edge, and walked across the rafters and ridge to the other side. Just then a big gust came through, lifting the plywood and its passenger off the roof. Larry said it was like parasailing, or at least what he imagined parasailing might be like. The wind carried him away about 200 feet, where he gradually descended and hit the ground with his feet under him. What a ride!

*   *   *

Another of the challenges of construction work is weather. Larry loved framing but wasn't so interested in the finish work that was done inside after all the walls were up, the roof on, and the windows and doors in. Colorado winters, however, discouraged most contractors from scheduling framing work between November and March. That's a big chunk of the year to be waiting for a paying job. Larry went back to stocking sheetrock in houses and apartments that were under construction. He typically lifted and carried two or three sheets at a time, but Tom recalls that sometimes they'd get in a hurry to finish and Larry would wet his gloves to improve his grip on the smooth paper covering, and carry four sheets at once. The apartments required 5/8" sheetrock because of the fire code for commercial buildings, and each 4' x 12' sheet weighed 135 pounds. The houses usually used 1/2" sheets of 112 pounds apiece. Obviously he had no need for a workout at the gym after days on a job like that!

One day while wrestling sheetrock up a tight stairwell, he lost his grip and the heavy sheets slipped and fell onto the top of Larry's left foot. Holy cow, did that hurt! The foreman told him to rest up for a day or two and get back to work as soon as he could; they needed him on this job. Well, Larry took a day off, used cold packs on his foot to help with the swelling, and then went back to his routine. Burl heard about it later and saw Larry's foot. He expressed the opinion that at least one of the bones that create the arch of the foot was broken. But no x-rays were taken, and no medical treatment addressed the issue. Years later, this would create or at least contribute to a problem.

A few years after Larry's parents divorced, Nadine had met and married John Muller. They'd moved to Springfield, Missouri, and the kids had all been to visit several times. Susan had married Ben Kuhn, and they'd made a fresh start for themselves in Springfield as well. Larry talked to Tom about the idea and they both agreed: "If you go, I'll go, too."

In 1973 the brothers moved to Missouri within two weeks of each other. They both found work at the Zenith plant, assembling televisions. There was still snow once in a while, but that didn't stop factory work. And the drifts never ever got up to the top four feet of the telephone poles like they'd seem 'em their last winter in Colorado.

*   *   *

Larry worked at Zenith for a couple of years and managed pretty well during that time. But the recession of the mid to late 1970s affected many jobs, and the trickle-down effect included fewer televisions being sold. Layoffs at the plant put him back on the street, looking for work. A constant issue for potential employers seemed to be Larry's diabetes. What if he had an insulin reaction while on the job? What if he hurt himself during one of those reactions, or even caused injury to someone else? No one wanted to be responsible for the potential liability issue such a scenario might create. At one point, pickings were so slim that Larry had taken up residence at the State Hotel in the older downtown district of Springfield. Originally built in 1906 as the Springfield Business College (with classes on the main floor and dormitory rooms above), the building had been converted to hotel use around 1918 and was in disrepair by the 1970s. Living there, however, was better than living on the street.

While residing in the State Hotel, Larry suffered another episode that nearly cost his life. Whether it was from too much insulin or too little, or simply from not enough food and no money to buy more, who knows? After not seeing him around the lobby for a couple of days, other residents of the hotel began to inquire of each other about Larry's whereabouts. Finally someone went upstairs to his door and knocked loudly several times. Through the transom window over the door they thought they could hear moaning inside, and the manager was summoned with the master key. Inside they found Larry on the floor, unconscious. An ambulance was called and he was transported to the nearest hospital, where he remained in a coma for almost two weeks. Finally, Larry woke up. The doctor treating him was amazed, and told him they'd just about given up hope.

"What is it here on Earth that's so important to you?" he asked. "Because it sure didn't look like you were going to stick around!"

Larry assured him there were plenty of things left for him to do, and that he had no intention of checking out so soon.

"I'm gonna live to be 100," he quipped.

Nadine was worried about him, though. She and John had an extra room at their house and insisted he come live with them. At least that way she could make sure he had enough to eat.

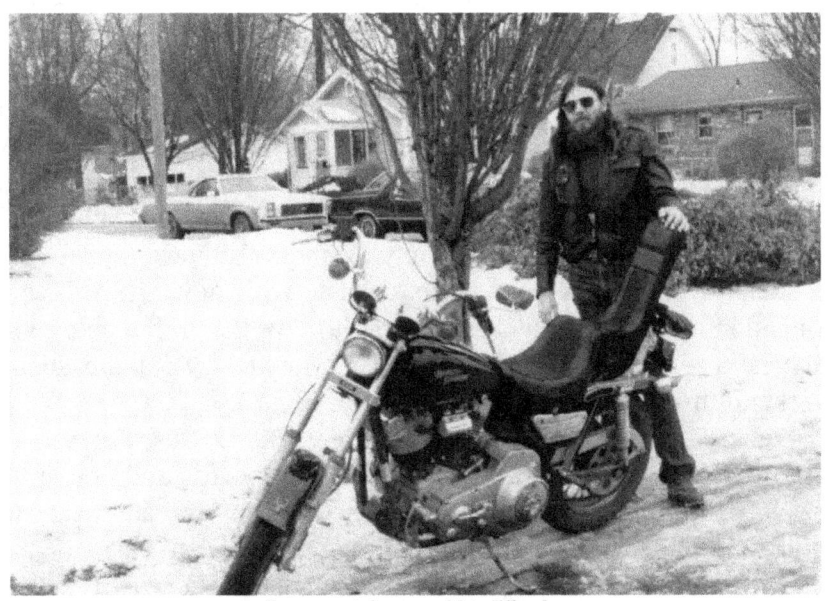

Larry with one of his Harleys

3
NOT A QUITTER

Over the next several years Larry worked a variety of jobs. He drove a cab for a while. He worked for his mom and stepdad John at their small appliance repair shop. An auto salvage yard kept him busy with a cutting torch, taking junk cars apart. One day the flame of the torch cut through Larry's right shoe and burned his foot. The fact that he didn't feel this happening right away was a sign of diabetic nephropathy; the disease was beginning to take a toll on the sensitivity of his nerve endings.

The burn was treated by a doctor more than once, but did not heal—maybe because Larry's diabetes was not well managed. Keep in mind that this was before home glucose monitors were available, and peeing on a special strip to test for ketones was the only option he had for checking how well his twice-daily insulin shots were controlling the disease. Maybe because Larry had no health insurance and couldn't afford the best doctors, or even the appropriate number of visits to an adequate doctor. Maybe it didn't help that he was still a smoker, and this restricted good blood flow to his feet. And maybe because he couldn't afford to stop working. At one point he went to University Hospital in Columbia, Missouri, for help. They tried using a skin graft to heal the wound. A social worker was sent in to consult with him. The doctors wanted him to stay off his feet in order to give the graft a chance to take hold and the burn an opportunity to mend. But the social worker didn't seem to have any ideas for him.

Larry went back to Springfield. By then he was working at Amos Millworks, a lumber company, lifting boards and operating a saw. The job had him on his feet 8 hours a day. To add insult to injury, his teeth had deteriorated severely (also due to the diabetes), and he'd finally had them all pulled. He would pack a lunch of scrambled egg sandwiches and applesauce or something else soft enough to gum, and put his feet up while he ate. Burl found out about this and sent enough money for Larry to have dentures made. Thank you, Dad!

But even the ability to chew couldn't help heal the open sore on his right foot, which began to turn dark. Larry felt sick a lot of the time, but continued to work as best he could. Finally the day came when he knew what had to be done. He sold his old car and bought a bus ticket for Columbia.

"I knew I wouldn't be driving when I came home," he told me later.

The doctors at University Hospital concurred; the foot had gangrene. The sickness was going to kill him if they didn't amputate. Larry told them he realized that, and it was why he was there.

The surgery was done and his right leg was removed about 4 inches below the knee. Within a few days the same social worker was sent in to see him.

"You again?" the guy sounded sarcastic and derisive. "I thought I told you before, there's nothing I can do to help you."

Larry stared at the man. How did a jerk like this ever get such a job? And why? What can you say in response to this kind of overt rudeness?

Without saying a word, Larry reached down and flipped back the covers from his abbreviated right leg, displaying the bandages over his stump.

"Oh, well, why didn't they say so? *Now* I can help you!"

And the social worker filled out the necessary paperwork to get Larry onto disability.

* * *

When the stitches were removed and there was no more sign of infection, the hospital dismissed Larry to go home and complete his recovery before getting a prosthetic leg. He had a pair of crutches and a list of exercises to do every day to keep the muscles in his upper leg strong and his knee joint flexible. The crutches, however, were awkward and difficult and his first day home one of them caught on something and he fell, landing directly on the stump of his right leg. The pain was excruciating, and it took him several minutes to get a deep breath and gather his strength to raise himself back up from the floor. He lived alone, but had reconciled

27

himself to doing whatever it took to make this work. Larry was not a quitter!

* * *

Without a car, he developed a routine of going to the little corner grocery down the road on his crutches and getting only a few items at a time. Observing this, the store owner asked if he could push a cart and use only one crutch; Larry tried it and succeeded.

"Ok, so get what you need, and take your bags home in the cart," the store owner said. "You can bring it back whenever you come, and leave it here when you get your new leg."

"But that'll be months," Larry told him.

"That's alright. I know you. You'll return it when you can," the owner said. And he was right.

Finally the day arrived for the return trip to Columbia. Larry was to stay at Rusk Rehabilitation Center—a part of the University Hospital system—while being fitted and trained to use his prosthesis.

Once the artificial limb was ready, the therapist showed him how to layer the special stump socks to achieve the right fit, helped him secure the leg with a heavy leather strap that clipped to a woven belt around his hips, and assisted Larry in standing up between a set of parallel bars.

"Now just stand still here for a minute if you can."

"But I want to *walk!*" Larry told him.

"I know, buddy, but you need to let your stump settle in and get used to the feel of the socket on that leg. It's probably going to hurt at first, and I don't want you to fall as soon as you put weight on it."

So they stood there for a minute or two.

"OK, now sit back down."

He did, and they relaxed for a few minutes.

"Now, do you want to try standing up with it by yourself?" the therapist asked.

"Yes."

"OK, I'll be right here if you start to wobble or feel weak."

"All right."

28

Larry took a deep breath and let it out slowly. He'd been practicing this over and over in his mind for months. He braced his arms on each side of the chair and stood up, grasping the bars ahead as he rose. Pausing just a second to assure the therapist he was steady, he took a step, then another.

"Now wait, you may not..." the therapist began.

"Man, let me do this. I know I can," Larry told him, and kept going. He had both hands on the bars but didn't need to put a lot of weight onto his arms. He'd been practicing those exercises religiously during the intervening months and was more than ready to move ahead.

When he reached the other end of the bars, he was careful and slowly made the turn to walk back to the other end. Another deliberate pivot, and he eased himself back into the waiting chair. Deep breath. Long exhale.

Larry looked up. "How was that?"

The therapist just grinned and shook his head. "I've never seen anyone do that well their first try. You're really something!"

"I'm determined," Larry told him. "This is not going to slow me down. I've got things to do. Someday I'm going to have a motorcycle again, and this new foot will have to control the brake. I'll have to take the test again to get my license, so I may as well start getting good with this thing now."

And he was well on his way.

* * *

During Larry's stay at Rusk, one of the nurses told him about Gary, a younger guy down the hall who'd had the same type of surgery Larry had had, but as a result of a motorcycle accident. Gary was also at Rusk to be fitted for a prosthetic leg, but was having a hard time with the mental/emotional part of his recovery. The nurse wanted to know if Larry would talk to him, try to impart some of his positive attitude to his fellow patient.

He said he'd try. By nature, Larry's personality was bashful and quiet. He much preferred to watch and listen to people than start a conversation, especially with someone he'd never met. But for the purpose of helping another, he screwed up his courage, knocked on the door, and entered the room down the hall.

He introduced himself to Gary, sat down in a chair by the bed, and told Gary the nurse had told him there was someone else on the floor who'd ridden bikes. Gary didn't ask why his visitor was a patient at Rusk, so Larry didn't mention it. They talked about motorcycles and places they'd ridden, where they were from, just general stuff.

Casually, Larry glanced over at the artificial leg propped up in the corner.

"So, how's it going with this thing?" he asked Gary.

"No good, man. It's just too hard. It really hurts." Gary's voice was full of discouragement.

"Yeah?" Larry continued, "They show you any exercises to do for muscle tone in that leg?"

"Yeah, I got a whole page of them things. I just hate doing 'em."

"Well, sure, but you gotta keep up with those to make this work, man." Larry was trying to keep the tone light, as he could tell this was a sensitive subject and didn't want to offend his new friend.

"Why bother?" Gary replied. "I'm done. I can't ride anymore, no girl's gonna want me like this, I may as well just give up right now."

"But..."

"No! Don't tell me how I gotta try and work and stuff like that; you don't know what it's like!" Gary was mad.

Larry sat still for a moment, letting Gary catch his breath and calm down. Then he slowly raised his hand and closed it into a loose fist. Keeping eye contact, he raised his right knee and lower leg, and used his knuckles to rap on the fiberglass prosthesis covered by his pant leg. It sounded like someone knocking at the door.

"Yeah, man, I do. I do know what it's like. It's not easy. It does hurt. You're right about that. But life's not over. You're still here, so there's gotta be a reason for that. We can't just give up. I *won't* give up. And I hope you won't, either."

Gary lowered his eyes. He could hear the sincerity in Larry's voice, but was struggling to get his head around this.

"I'll think about it," he finally said.

"OK," Larry replied. "That's good enough for me... for now."

He smiled and said goodnight, then got up and walked back to his room down the hall. Gary noticed that he didn't even seem to limp.

The next morning, when Larry was in physical therapy, Gary arrived in his wheelchair, his prosthesis balanced across his lap.

"You're early!" the therapist exclaimed; usually they had to go coax Gary out of bed to even get him as far as the chair.

Gary gave a slight smile and motioned to Larry. "Yeah, this guy here gave me a pep talk last night. I thought about it, and decided he may be right. I need to at least try to make this work. Maybe if I can see how he does it..."

So they worked together, the two bikers and the therapists. Before too many days went by, the guys were laughing together and competing to see who could walk the farthest or the fastest or with the most natural gait. And when they weren't wearing their prostheses, they had wheelchair races down the long, straight hallways or outside on the sidewalks. Larry had learned how to pop "wheelies" in the wheelchair, and taught Gary how to do this without tipping the chair over backward. Some watching patients were amused, but the nurses were scared (almost) speechless.

Life was not over for either of them.

4
A DREAM COME TRUE

June 1983

I'd moved again. For 4 years it had seemed like I was almost always moving. This was a relative thing, since I had spent my first (almost) 18 years living in one house, where my parents are still living now. In August 1979, I'd moved into a dorm room in Springfield, Missouri, to start college. By January 1980 I'd moved down the hall to get a private room in a suite with four other girls instead of five. Four months later, I moved back home for the summer, only to repeat the same pattern over the next 12 months. In August 1981 my folks helped me locate a tiny two-room apartment on the second floor of an old house that had been converted to student housing. There were two other miniscule apartments for female students upstairs, and all second-floor tenants shared the bathroom at the top of the stairs that looked so decrepit we were sure it had come over on the Ark. Or at least the Mayflower. I'd stayed in the apartment my final 2 years of school, but now that was done. Graduated! I had no idea where life would take me, but I was ready to find out. I'd started kindergarten at age 4 (almost 5) and was now 21; it seemed like I'd been in school *forever.*

My friend Tammy's mom worked at a credit union that owned some rental property, and a duplex apartment had come open. It was actually another older house that had been divided into two apartments, but this one was in much better shape and had more space. There was a small living room and a large kitchen with room for a table, chairs, and a washer/dryer set that Tammy's dad supplied and installed so we needn't sit around at the laundromat to do our laundry. The bathroom was blessedly modern, and there were three bedrooms, one each for Tammy, our mutual friend Lisa, and myself. We each paid $87 a month, which included utilities, trash service, and lawn care—not a bad deal in 1983! We could all cook, and we took turns with kitchen duties. Tammy was the only one of us with a boyfriend at the time, but Randy had his own place. Friends would drop by to visit, and we'd occasionally go out to dinner or a movie. Lisa and Tammy both had jobs in the public library system, and I was On The Hunt. I checked ads in the paper, went to the Job Service office, and by August 8 I was employed by the company I still work for now.

But in the meantime, not long after the girls and I moved in to our bachelorette pad, I met Larry.

The duplex faced south toward Cherry Street, and the front porch was just outside our living room. I'd planted flowers in front of the house the day before; impatiens in front of the porch, with purple and yellow petunias alternating along the base of the front wall of the adjoining apartment. I'd checked with Steve, the tenant there, before planting anything on his side, and he didn't mind.

Lisa and I were in the living room with the main door open to let air through the screen door, when I heard the sound of a motorcycle approaching, slowing, turning into the driveway of our abode, and then finally coasting to a stop just south of Steve's living room, which extended out farther than ours, the width of the front porch. The rider took off his helmet to reveal light brown hair pulled back into a short, wavy ponytail. His long slim legs were nicely displayed in snug Levi boot jeans (30 × 36 I found out later!). A handsome face, lean muscular arms, long mustache, sideburns, sunglasses. *Man*, did he look cool.

"Oh, I could fall for that," I thought. "Probably not a good idea, though; he looks like the kind who could break my heart." I'd had a couple of somewhat serious boyfriends, but obviously none who had worked out long term. But hey, I was 21!

So I stepped out through the screen door, planted my feet at the edge of the porch, stood with my hands on my hips, and asked the biker: "Did you run over my flowers?!"

He looked up at me from under a somewhat lowered brow. "No."

Hmm. Not such a good start.

"What kind of chopper is that?"

"BSA."

"What year?"

"It's a '68."

"Oh. So, how's it run?"

Again, the heavy brows weren't in the friendliest position... "How do you think?"

Apparently Larry had just recently purchased this motorcycle from a little shop downtown and was finding it a challenge to keep it running. He told me that all afternoon he'd been messing with it. Ride 15 minutes, stop and work on it for 30. Ride 10 minutes, monkey with it 45. Not the type of day to put someone in the best of moods, and then when he's just minding his own business, going to visit his old friend Steve, here's this girl he's never met, accusing him of running over her flowers!

Somehow we managed to exchange names, and I planted the seed that I wouldn't mind a ride if he ever got the bike running right. He seemed to consider this, but no promises were made.

* * *

September 9, 1983

Larry had been in Colorado for the past month. The BSA chopper had been swapped back to the shop back in June, after 3 weeks of continuous problems, and the 1978 Triumph Bonneville 750cc bike he'd gotten to replace it ran a lot better. He'd made a road trip to visit his family back home with the intention of staying a couple of weeks, but had such a good time he ended up staying longer. His dad tried to talk him into moving back to Colorado Springs, and mentioned the idea of classes at the community college there to help him learn a trade that didn't require a lot of time on his feet. Burl also asked Larry something along the lines of, "Don't you think it's about time you settled down and started a family?" After all, he was pushing 34. Larry admitted there was a girl he'd met back in Missouri who had him considering his options. But he'd been alone a long time—9 years, in fact. Two previous attachments had left him emotionally bruised and more wary than ever.

But now he was back in Missouri, sitting in Steve's living room in Springfield. He heard footsteps on the front porch; it was the

34

girls next door, returning home from somewhere.

"Man, my neighbor's been asking about you. Wondering when you were coming back from out west," Steve told him.

Larry didn't have to ask which neighbor he meant. We'd talked a few times during the summer when he came by to visit Steve. A couple times I'd hinted about that bike ride I wanted, and at least once he'd responded with "What are you doing tomorrow?" but I'd already had plans. What he didn't mention to Steve (and didn't tell me for quite a while) was that he'd seen me before we'd ever met over the flowers outside, in a dream he'd had earlier that year.

In the dream he was riding his motorcycle and wound around through some hills down to a rocky riverside, where I was standing near the water. He found a piece of paper on the ground—a flyer about an event or something—and asked me about it. Details were fuzzy, but by the end of the dream we were both on the motorcycle, riding away. That's all he recalled.

As Lisa and I arrived home that evening the motorcycle parked in the driveway caught my eye immediately. *"Larry's back!"* I realized. It seemed like he'd been gone a long time, and I didn't waste too many moments in our duplex before stepping over to Steve's door. I sat on the sofa near Larry and heard all about his trip to Colorado, and told him about the job I'd started the month before. We talked about the mountains, about riding motorcycles, about Native Americans (he liked turquoise jewelry as much as I did)... on and on. At one point I looked across the living room at their friends Tom and Christine, who had also dropped by to visit, and saw them staring wide-eyed at the two of us.

"What?" I asked.

"We're just fascinated to see Larry actually *talking* to someone," Christine said.

Tom said something about usually needing a prybar to get two words out of Larry. Steve just smiled.

Next thing I knew it was after 1 am.

"Well" I said to Larry, "I can see right now I'm going to have to pin you down on when you're going to take me for that bike ride, before you go off on another month-long road trip!"

"How about tomorrow?" he asked.

I groaned. "I'm leaving in the morning for St Louis. Have a wedding to go to. In fact I need to get up at 5 to leave on time."

"When are you coming back?"

"Sunday evening."

"What time?"

"Probably 8 PM or so."

"I'll be here by 9," he said.

And he was. We went for an evening ride on Sunday, September 11, 1983. It was our first date, and my 22nd birthday. We were virtually inseparable afterward.

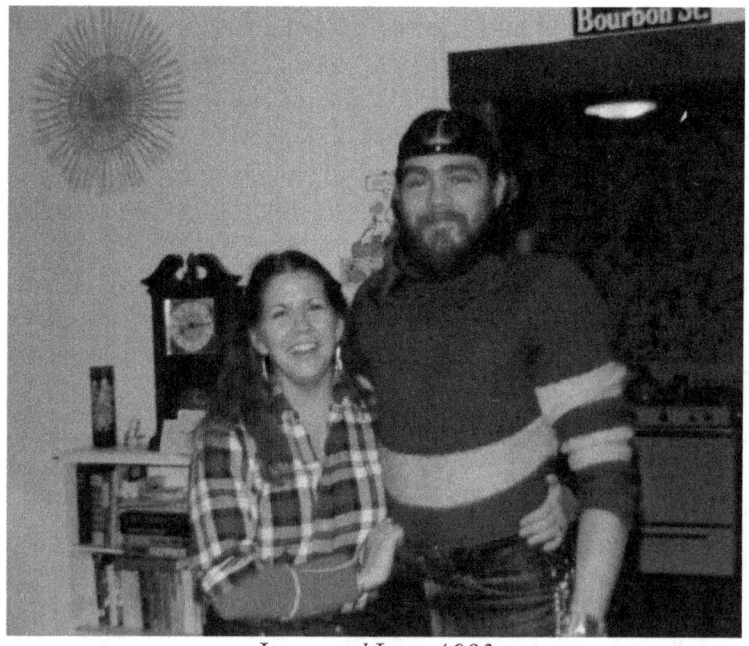

Larry and Jesse, 1983

5
DETERMINED

One of the guys who hung out around Steve's place had told me Larry had an artificial leg. It didn't bother me. Larry probably told me himself he had gotten diabetes at a very early age. I knew so little about the disease that I wasn't scared by that either. The fact that he was 12 years older than me, unemployed (on disability), and rode a motorcycle prompted my dad to advise me to "drop him like a hot potato," but I was not dissuaded.

We dated regularly that autumn. Before Christmas we were seriously committed. I took him home to meet my folks the weekend after Valentine's Day, 1984. They treated him kindly, and he'd won them both over before we left. We married March 24 and started settling in to a little rental house a couple of blocks from the duplex where we'd met.

By then I'd experienced one major insulin reaction in Larry. At first I hadn't known that's what it was; all I knew was that Larry had gotten quiet and then simply quit talking to me. About the time I was getting insulted and upset about this, he "came to" enough to tell me he was having a low-sugar episode and needed something to eat. Some orange juice and a few slices of cinnamon toast later, he was sufficiently back to normal to tell me the story behind the "no glass glasses during a reaction" rule. As time went on I learned to watch for signs that his blood sugar was dipping too low: abnormal sweating, inappropriate sleepiness, twitchy muscles, incomplete and/or nonsensical sentences... sometimes I saw only one of these things, sometimes all, and sometimes none. If an insulin reaction occurred during the day, Larry could often feel himself "getting low" and would eat something to counteract it. In November 1983 he'd received his first blood glucose testing meter for home use, and in addition to regular testing in the mornings and evenings, this machine could help confirm or deny a suspected reaction. I learned to be especially sensitive to any abnormal sounds or movements he might make in the night, since a drop in blood sugar during sleep can quickly progress to a critical (perhaps even fatal) stage without the sufferer feeling it.

Low blood sugar events are hard on diabetic patients. Although juice, soda, or sweet treats might help them regain lost ground on the glucose "mountain," it can also send them to the top of a slippery slope that can have them plummeting just as fast down the other side again if the remedial snack isn't followed up with something that will hold them a little longer, such as a sandwich, eggs and toast, cheese and crackers, or apple wedges and peanut butter. Even then, a bad reaction can still result in side effects such as chills, headache, exhaustion, or a general feeling of weakness that may last several hours. Larry often had these physical issues, and although he didn't talk about it much, I knew there were emotional side effects as well. He hated the feeling that he'd been out of control, of not remembering what might have just happened, of being what he called "lost in the forest." Likewise, those same events are difficult for the diabetic's family. More than once over the coming years I would deal with severe insulin reactions that had Larry in a state of confusion, and some of them got a little ugly. During nighttime reactions it wasn't unusual for Larry to just roll over and cover his head, cocooning himself in the perceived safety of the darkness as I tried to rouse him enough to consume something with the necessary carbohydrates to bring him back around. A couple of times when I offered the plastic cup of juice or Pepsi to begin bringing him back up from "The Depths," he became disoriented or irritated enough to flail out with an arm, sometimes knocking the cup from my hands and making a sticky mess of us and everything nearby in the process. At least once he struck me in the face during an episode like this. Of course I cried out rather loudly at that, and then Larry's eyes popped open and he realized what he'd done and was absolutely horrified. Warrior spirit, yes—but he would *never* intentionally hit a woman. One night years later, after we'd moved to a farmhouse where our bedroom was upstairs, Larry was so discombobulated by the low blood sugar that when trying to lose himself in the quilts didn't get me to leave him alone, he got up out of the bed and made his way out into the hallway (without his prosthetic leg), where he tried to climb over the railing that surrounded the stairwell. It took some quick maneuvering and fast talking to prevent that one from going very bad! After nights like these I was physically, mentally, and emotionally exhausted, too. And unlike him, I had to get up and go to work the next morning.

*   *   *

Who was it who said, "Life is what happens while you're busy making other plans"? As I mentioned earlier, we began to set up housekeeping together in a rental house just after our wedding. Larry still had some things in the tiny house he had been renting before that on Nettleton Avenue, and I still had stuff in the duplex on Cherry Street when life threw us a curve on April 18, 1984.

It was a Wednesday night. I'd worked that day, and then we took a short ride on the Triumph, stopping at a pharmacy to get more test strips for the glucose meter, followed by supper at a cafeteria on Glenstone Avenue, and then we headed home. It was dark, but this was the main street in town, there were streetlights everywhere, and we didn't have far to go. And yes, the headlight was on, and the bike—while not a Harley—was loud. But as we approached a green light at the corner of Glenstone and Cherry, the driver of a station wagon coming in the opposite direction apparently didn't see us and made a left turn directly into our path.

I was looking at the stores off to our left. Larry made some sort of sound that caused me to look forward. I thought, "This is it. This is the one we're not going to get out of." Then BOOM. I was propelled ass-over-appetite into the air, over the top of the station wagon and into the oncoming lane of traffic. Larry, who couldn't very well take an evasive "tuck & roll" measure with me on the back, had done everything he could to stop, but the bike struck the right side of the station wagon hard, throwing him forward. His helmet broke the passenger side center window. He had braked and downshifted so hard the pedals for those controls were bent down, almost under the motorcycle. There was 23 feet of skidmark on the pavement. The front wheel was pushed backward into the motor, and the handlebars were bent forward from the impact of his hips.

Neither of us was knocked unconscious, though, and when the

39

spinning stopped I looked around for Larry. At the same time he sat up and called desperately for me, trying to figure out where I was. Then the pain hit and he groaned and collapsed back down onto the asphalt. Thank God the oncoming traffic had stopped and I wasn't hit. I scrambled up and ran back to Larry. Incredibly the Triumph, laying there on its left side, was still running and he asked me turn off the key to shut down the motor. Soon an ambulance showed up and took us to the hospital. The occupants of the station wagon were unhurt.

The doctors there diagnosed Larry with a broken bone in his right forearm and five breaks in his pelvis. They also said that because of the impact to his private parts he might be sterile. He stayed in ICU for a few days, and then was moved to a room where they rigged a trapeze bar over the bed so he could grasp it with his left hand to help move himself when he needed to reposition. An orthopedic surgeon put a plate in his right arm because there was a little chip out of the bone (we never did know where it went!) but said the pelvic fractures would just take time.

They tried to prepare us for what to expect.

"Two to three months before you'll walk alone again," the doctor told Larry, "and I'll have the physical therapy department rig up a brace on the right side of a walker for you to rest your cast."

Larry was truly bummed. We weren't even done moving yet! And (again, thank God!) we had a baby on the way. He was determined this setback was not going to keep him down for long. We had the prayer support of both of our families and many friends, and he was going to surpass the expectations of the doctors and the therapists, or know the reason why.

Exactly 3 weeks after the accident, he went to physical therapy for the first time. Two therapists were ready to work with him and helped him put on his prosthesis. With one on each side, they levered an arm under each of his armpits and helped him to stand up from the wheelchair at one end of a set of parallel bars.

"Steady now, just try standing still here for a minute," one therapist told him. "If you start to get dizzy, tell us, and we'll sit you back down."

40

So they stood. One minute, then two.

"Now what?" Larry asked.

"How about trying a step?" the lead therapist quizzed.

"Sure," was the reply.

So they moved a step forward, all three of them, the therapists still helping to support Larry closely from each side. Then another step, and another. By the time they reached the other end of the parallel bars and helped him turn around, Larry said he thought one helper was enough. After a few more steps he offered to try it alone. They didn't move far off, but did turn him loose to watch him finish the walk back toward the chair.

"OK! Are you ready to sit down then?"

"No, I want to walk some more." Larry told them. "Can you please move that chair? I don't think I need these bars."

"Don't you think you've done enough for your first day?" one of them asked.

Larry smiled and asked her again to move the chair.

The lead therapist brought a four-footed cane with a stout handle, contoured for steady gripping.

"Here, try this, and stay close to the wall where there's a rail you can grab if you need it. I know your right arm's in that cast, but we'll be right behind you with the chair if you need to sit down."

They started walking the perimeter of the room. When the square was complete, the therapist had a lighter cane, the "normal" style without the four-footed base.

"Want to try this one?"

"Yeah."

"Sure you're not too tired?"

"No, thanks."

And another circuit was made. By this time the second therapist had beckoned to some nurses and other staff from the doorway, and there was a bit of an audience hovering around the entry to the physical therapy room, watching his steps. Whispers were exchanged about this being Larry's first visit to the room since his motorcycle accident 3 weeks before, and how all four of the small bones that meet at the middle of the pelvis were broken, one of them in two places.

As he approached the group by the door, Larry handed off the cane to the therapist.

"You can have this back," he told her with a smile. "I don't think I need it after all." And he kept on walking.

The next day the doctor heard about this and came to the therapy room to see for himself. The day after that he let Larry come home.

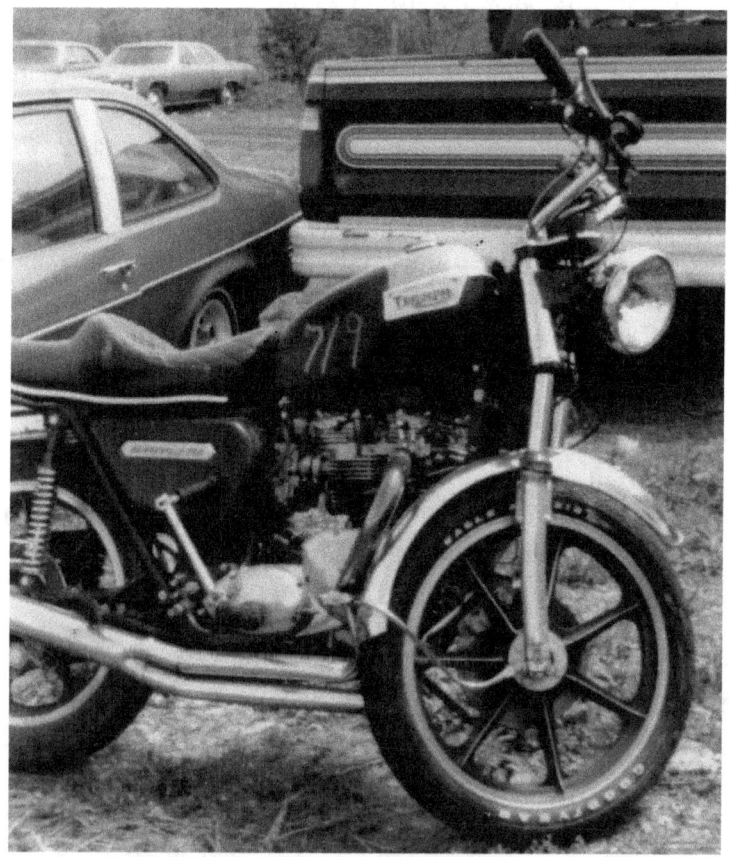

1978 Triumph 750 Bonneville

6
FIGHTING TO STAY AFOOT

Daddy's Little Princess was named Jennifer Lynn. Larry had told me he wanted a girl and that we were going to have a girl. My mother also believed we'd be having a girl (their first grandchild!). Me? I didn't have a strong feeling about it one way or the other, and I was *carrying* this child!

One day we were talking about baby names. We'd finally narrowed it down to a couple of possibilities on the Girl list, then decided we'd have to actually see her first before the final decision.

"OK, so now what about Boy names?" I asked.

"What about 'em?" was Larry's response.

"Well, we need to pick a couple of those, too." I ventured.

"No, we don't." he said. "We're not having a boy."

"What makes you so sure?"

"I just know," he nodded.

And apparently, he did.

By now the cast was off his arm and Larry was moving around pretty well. His right hand would never again pivot over flat with the palm up—making it difficult to accept change back from a clerk, for instance—but he had a good grip and could use the arm. And he could walk just as well as before, and without a cane. People who didn't know him and even most of our casual acquaintances had no idea he wore a prosthetic leg, because he worked hard to walk without a limp.

Before the motorcycle accident Larry had talked to an occupational therapist about getting some training and trying to get back to work. That plan was derailed by his long recuperation, and now we had a baby at home. It had never been my dream to have a career instead of staying home with my child, but life can be pretty ironic. At least when I went back to the office I had the assurance that Jennifer's daddy would take every bit as much care with her as

I would. We lived close enough to my place of employment that I went home at lunchtime, allowing me to feed Jennifer and make sure Larry was eating, too.

*　　*　　*

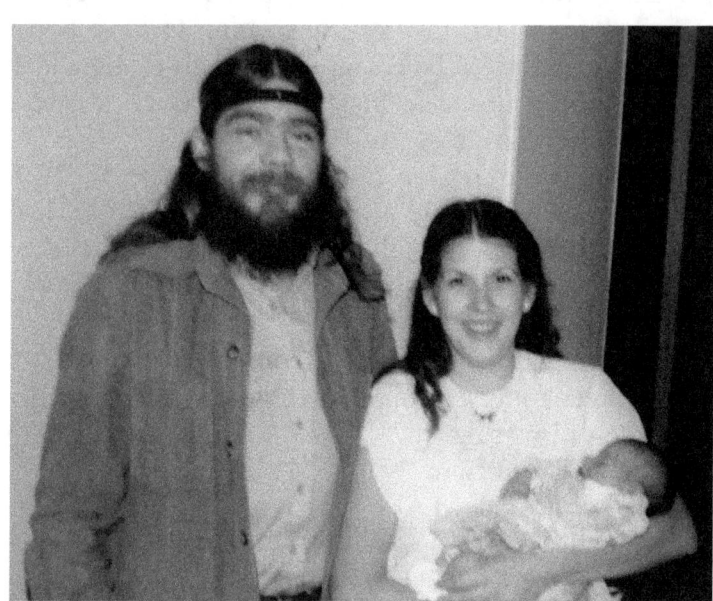

October, 1984

When we met, Larry had already suffered the amputation of his right leg below the knee, and was battling a sore on the bottom of his left foot that just wouldn't heal. He'd spent several days in the hospital because of it during the November we were dating, but nothing seemed to help much. The ulcer was about 1 to 2 inches in diameter at any given time, and at least 1/2 inch deep. The fact that he wasn't standing on concrete 8 hours a day, as he had at many of his former jobs, didn't seem to make a difference. That sore was stubborn! He took his insulin and kept his foot clean and protected. The doctors said it had to heal from the inside out and that until the gap filled in, there wasn't much point in doing a skin graft.

In March 1985 Larry became ill with what seemed like flu symptoms: fever, nausea, fatigue, general malaise. I had called his doctor's office that first day, but was told it was probably just something that was going around, to make sure his blood sugar stayed in control, and to try to keep him hydrated.

I can't remember if he'd been in bed two days or three when he commented, "It's probably my foot."

"What do you mean?" I asked.

Larry pulled back the covers at the lower edge of the bed and showed me his left foot, which now had a bulging shiny spot near the inside of the foot, at the top, directly above the ulcer on the bottom. The skin over this spot was thin and translucent, and whatever was underneath it looked very dark, almost black.

"That's how it started when my right foot went bad," he told me.

I went into orbit.

Immediately, I called the doctor's office. He was out of town, something about a golf tournament. (They probably weren't supposed to tell me that!) As politely as I could, I conveyed to the receptionist the sense of urgency I felt this situation deserved. She managed to juggle the schedule and make an appointment for Larry to see the doctor who was on call that day. He took one look at Larry's foot and sent us to the hospital.

"That needs surgery!" he told us. "The wound needs to be cleaned out, and you'll need IV antibiotics to help get rid of that infection. You might lose that foot, too."

As it turned out, surgery was the best possible answer, because they found a bone spur on the bottom of Larry's foot that was contributing to the ulcer. The surgeon shaved the spur down while he was cleaning out the nasty stuff, and the bottom of the foot actually healed up before the top!

But the cleanout was extensive, all the way from the top of his foot down through the bottom, and again we were told that it would need to heal from the inside out. Larry was on two strong antibiotics, one given every 4 hours and the other given every 6 hours, around the clock. The wound was cleaned twice a day and loosely packed with gauze soaked in a special solution to promote the growth of new, healthy tissue.

After several days of this, he started feeling well enough to be getting bored in the hospital.

"Why can't I be doing this at home?" he quizzed the doctor one morning when rounds were made.

"Because of the IV meds," the doctor said.

"We could do those at home," Larry argued.

"Oh, we can't allow that, that's a very technical process and the drugs have to be administered at a certain rate on a very strict schedule," was the response.

Larry wasn't deterred. "I've been watching what the nurses do when they come in here. I see where they set the regulator and I can tell you exactly how many seconds go by between the drops from that bag. If you tell me the schedule I *promise* I will stick to it. I am going NUTS in here, man. You gotta let me go home!"

Whether it was Larry's sincerity or the pleading look in his eyes, the doctor was convinced... but only so far. He arranged for the bandages, solutions, equipment, and medications to be sent home with us. I received training in cleaning and dressing the wound. They showed us both how to hook up the IV for the antibiotics, how to flush the IV port before and after with saline, and how to put in the heparin lock to keep it from clotting up. But the doctor would approve only one of the medications to go home with us: the one that was dosed every 6 hours. We figured if we ran it on the 6s and 12s we'd be sure to keep the schedule straight. It took about 30 minutes to run the full dose, so it made for a short night, but we managed.

After a week we returned to the doctor's office for a status check. Not good. There was pus in the wound.

Back to the hospital. Larry was put in an isolation room where no visitors were allowed without covering up in blue hospital garb, including booties and a mask. Until they could culture the stuff and the lab could figure out exactly what sort of bacteria was causing the problem, they weren't taking any chances.

And that's how we spent our first wedding anniversary.

Finally the report was in, and the doctor confirmed that while Larry didn't have to stay in the hospital, he really did need to stay

46

on that second antibiotic. Instead of every 4 hours, though, we'd administer it every 8 hours, in addition to the other one every 6 hours. The two medicines could be run together, so we devised a new schedule. The 6 am dose would include both drugs. I'd run the single dose at noon when I was home for lunch. A visiting nurse would come by at 2 pm each day to deliver the second dose of the high-powered stuff and do a wound check, and the 6 pm, 10 pm, and midnight rounds we'd handle ourselves. The hospital pharmacy made up enough IV bags for 5 days' worth of treatment at a time. One day's doses were kept in the refrigerator, and the rest stayed in the freezer. Every night I transferred the following day's bags into the refrigerator to thaw, and every fifth day I went by the hospital to pick up more antibiotics. Every week we saw the doctor.

It was hectic, but it worked! After just 3 weeks, the ulcer that had been on the bottom of Larry's foot for 2 to 3 years was finally healed. The top took several weeks longer, but the infection was cleared, and the hole eventually closed up. No skin graft was required.

Hallelujah!

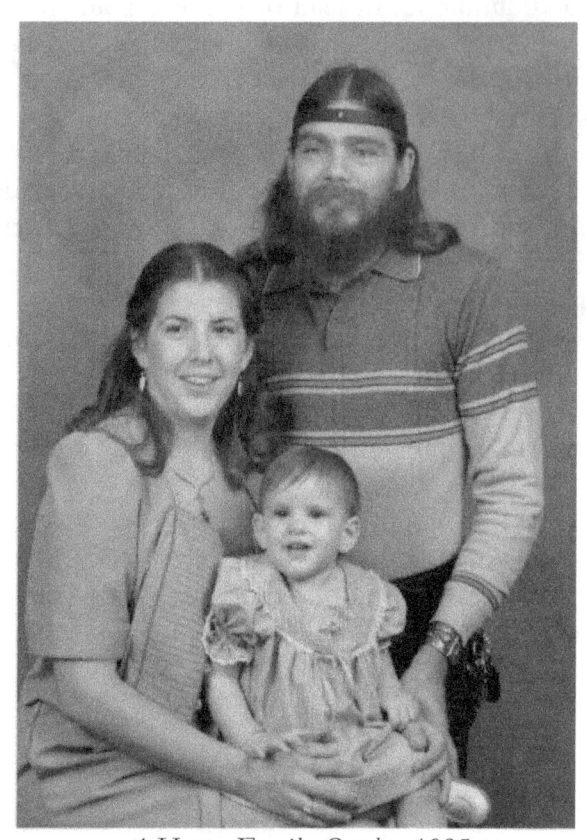

A Happy Family, October 1985

7
WELCOME HOME

Fall, 1992

Our daughter Jennifer was starting second grade. The little house we'd bought after 4 years of renting was within walking distance of her grade school, in a quiet neighborhood with mature trees. It was a nice enough place to live, but I'd always had the dream of living in the country. I wanted *land.* Larry liked the conveniences of town but raised show pigeons as a hobby. This apparently caused concern for the little old lady next door, who complained to the city, which sent us a letter citing an ordinance regarding "poultry." I showed the letter to my boss—who also happened to be an attorney—and explained that we didn't consider pigeons to be poultry, that we didn't let them fly over her house or roost on her gutters or poop on her patio. The birds had a little shed with an attached "flight pen" made of wood framing and completely covered by chicken wire. They were not allowed out of those enclosures. He recommended a personal visit with the neighbor to smooth things over, and we did that. But the initial trust and feelings of goodwill had been broken, and we never again felt truly comfortable there. If I worked in my little vegetable garden out back, there she'd be, peeking through her window curtains at me. When Larry cleaned the little pigeon coop, she found reasons to trim her hedge or prune her flowers or something else out back that would put her in a prime position to throw out a little comment or two.

We needed to move.

The answer came that fall, with a "move out to move up" situation through my employer. A smaller branch office about 110 miles north of Springfield in Sedalia had an opening for an office adjuster, working smaller insurance claims that could be handled over the phone, through the mail, or directly with clients who had drivable vehicles and were able to come by the branch office for inspection. I applied, was interviewed, and got the job. The company even paid for the move!

I found a real estate agent to help me look for just the right property. She knew we wanted a place with 10 acres or more, a barn or shed for Larry's pigeons, and a basement, and that we preferred a two-story house. It took some looking, and we ended up 20 miles from my new office, but what we finally found seemed perfect: 50 acres, an old farmhouse probably built in the 1920s, with bedrooms upstairs, the requisite basement with an overhead door so Larry's motorcycle could be parked inside, a big old hay barn with a 20 x 30 dairy barn on the east side and a 3-stall lean-to on the west, plus a little tack barn with 2 box stalls in the corral close to the house. The milk barn was the optimal spot for Larry's pigeons, and he immediately set about creating pens and nesting boxes. Our land stretched west and north from the house. To our east was crop land, and no other house for a mile. Across the road to the south was pasture land with a creek running through it. The roads near the house were (and still are) gravel, and it was 8 or 9 miles (depending on which route you drove) into the little town where Jennifer would go to school, but we were thrilled. At last... space to breathe.

*   *   *

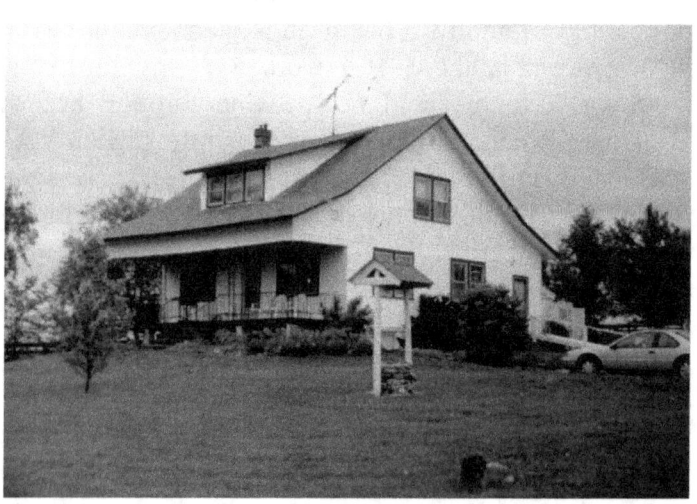

Farmhouse

Winter 1992–1993

We'd moved to the farm in October. My folks were going to come for Thanksgiving weekend—their first view of our little piece of the earth, and I was really looking forward to it. The Wednesday night beforehand I left work as soon as the office closed at 4:30, put gas in the car, took books back to the library, made a last-minute stop at the grocery with the hordes of other folks getting ingredients for their holiday meals, and headed for home. The days were short enough that this many errands meant I was driving home in the dark. Another aspect of country living that hadn't really sunk in with me yet was the abundance of deer in the vicinity, and that harvest season meant combines and grain trucks in the fields, and how that combination along with mating season meant lots of deer running amok all over the place.

You can guess what happened next.

Ever noticed how deer will see a vehicle's lights coming, hear the engine's noise, and still just jump right out in front of it? Well, nobody ever said they were the smartest animal in the world.

Missouri Highway 52 is two lanes wide. That's it. No shoulders, no passing lanes, no extra pavement whatsoever. When the deer jumped up out of the ditch to my right, I had the briefest glimpse of it before it collided with the front end of the little Ford Tempo I was driving. I'm not sure I even had time to hit the brakes before it was over and the deer flew off into the opposite ditch and I slowed to a stop at the side of the road. The car was still running and didn't appear to be leaking any fluid. I still had one good headlight and wasn't hurt, so I drove on home.

It shook me up a little and cost me the deductible on my insurance, but I learned a valuable lesson. *Watch Out For Deer!*

The car had been fixed for maybe 4 or 5 weeks when the weather turned ugly around the 20th of January, giving us 2 to 3 inches of snow on the ground and then frosting that cake with about a 1/2-inch of ice and sleet. I'd driven in snow a little, but not nearly as much as Larry had. Still, I had a job to get to and thought I could handle it. After all, the snow wasn't deep.

Our house is about 3 miles from the nearest paved road. I made it to within a quarter mile of good ol' Highway 52 when the car started to fishtail on the slick road. Unable to bring it back into control, I could only hold on as it headed for the ditch on the west side. "Jesus, help me!" I called out.

The Tempo went nose down, then wheels up, then down on the roof in the grassy ditch, with the wheels still turning like a stranded turtle, trying to paddle its way back to mobility. I unhooked my seatbelt, hunted around for my purse and crawled out the broken window. Amazingly I was not hurt. Embarrassed and shook up (again), but not hurt. I started walking toward home. A neighbor came by in his truck and gave me a ride home.

Jennifer was getting ready for school upstairs; her bedroom windows overlooked the driveway. She heard the truck and peeked outside.

"Daddy, there's a truck outside... and Mama's getting out of it!" she called down to Larry.

Larry thought to himself: "Oh, she's probably slid the car off into the ditch. I'll have to take a chain and pull it out with the pickup."

The pickup wasn't the machine for the job, though. A wrecker had to go get it, and this time the little Tempo wouldn't fix.

*   *   *

February 1993

In the Big List of Stressors we deal with throughout life, choosing a car should rank fairly high up the list, or at least it should on my list. I'm a creature of habit, I'll admit it. I've been known the carry the same purse for a year or more until it's coming apart, then finally pick another one I think will work, then wait another 3 months before ever transferring the items from the old purse to the new one. Some of us really resist change.

After the Tempo was totaled by the big flip into the ditch, we couldn't waste a lot of time making a choice on a car. Larry used his pickup to take Jennifer to school every morning and pick her up every afternoon (he'd heard horror stories about how some kids act on the bus and didn't want her exposed to that). So we made the rounds of the car lots.

52

A lot of looking and a few test drives later, we bought a 1992 Ford Thunderbird. It was a pretty teal color called Cayman Green, and had only 3,778 miles on the odometer, making it the newest car either of us had ever owned. Unfortunately we didn't own it very long. In fact, it lasted 30 days.

On Saturday, February 27, Larry took the list of errands to be done and headed out in the T-bird. His truck was in the shop, getting the motor for the heater fan replaced. Jennifer almost always went along with her daddy, but since I was baking chocolate chip cookies she elected to stay home and help.

Larry stopped by the propane office in Windsor and paid the bill for the fill-up they'd done earlier in the week. He went by the bank and got some money out of savings as I'd requested. He filled the gas tank in the car. The next stop was in Clinton, 25 miles southwest of home, where he picked up four 50-pound bags of specialty feed for his show pigeons. The list was done, and it was time to head home.

But just a few miles east of Clinton something happened. Was it an insulin reaction? A mini-stroke? A dropped cigarette that had him looking down? We'll never know, but the end result was that he crossed the center line into the opposite lane. An oncoming car took to the shoulder of the road to avoid hitting him. The next car veered into the eastbound lane instead of the shoulder, just about the time the Thunderbird headed back that way. WHAM!

It was bad. The driver of the other car was picked up by friends and sought treatment for back problems later. Because he hired an attorney right away, we were not given the details of his injury, and our insurance company settled the claim. But the ambulance personnel and the highway patrol had to call for the Jaws of Life to pry open the T-bird and extricate Larry. The hood looked more like a triangle shape than a square, with the left front being pushed in and back. The left front wheel had been driven back almost to the driver's seat. Our new car was mangled, and so was Larry.

The police called to let me know about the accident and to tell me that Larry had been taken by ambulance to Golden Valley Medical Center in Clinton, but was being airlifted to Research Medical Center in Kansas City, about 100 miles northwest of us.

His injuries were very serious.

With the truck still in the shop, I had no transportation, and called my friend and co-worker Kay Smith. She dropped everything and came 25 miles south from LaMonte to pick up Jennifer and me and drive us to Research. Before we left home I'd called my cousin Jeff, who lived near the hospital, and my parents. We were all pretty scared, not knowing what we'd hear when we got there.

Jeffrey was there waiting when Jennifer, Kay, and I walked in to the ER. My brother David had called from Tennessee, and Jeff was on the phone in the waiting room, answering any questions that he could for David and his wife Abby. A nurse had given Jeff a plastic bag with Larry's rings and the silver, ebony, and turquoise bracelet I'd bought for him on his first Father's Day. Jeff told me they were getting Larry ready for surgery. He had several broken bones and a "belly full of blood," they'd said.

A nurse took me back to the cubicle where Larry was on a gurney. He was covered from toes to neck with sheets and blankets. They must've given him plenty of pain medication, as he didn't appear to be in any great discomfort. He was conscious and knew me on sight. I'm not sure he fully realized where he was, however, and if so, he certainly didn't recall why. I stroked his face and talked to him for just a minute when the nurse came in to tell me they were ready to go. I bent to kiss Larry and told him I'd be there when he got back.

"Where am I going?" he asked.

"To surgery," the nurse and I both told him.

"Why?"

"Because you're hurt," I replied. "You were in an accident."

"I *was?*" He was incredulous.

"Yes." I nodded. "In the new car."

Larry frowned at that. He almost always drove his old orange Chevy pickup. The Great Pumpkin, I called it.

"You were running errands and had a bad car accident on your way home from Clinton."

A look of horror and fear crossed his features.

"Where's Jennifer? Is Jennifer OK?" He was panicking now.

Even if his short-term memory had been affected by the blow to his head, his instincts about her, and especially about her almost always being with him, were intact.

"Jennifer's fine. She was home with me. We baked cookies." I smiled to reassure him.

"Oh. OK. That's good then."

The nurse indicated that they really needed to go.

"Love you," I smiled again and gave him a quick kiss on the lips.

"I love you, too," he said, and they wheeled him away.

The surgery—or surgeries, rather—lasted about 9-1/2 hours. First the trauma surgeon opened his belly area and repaired a lacerated liver and a lacerated spleen. They also found a vein that had torn loose and was causing the massive internal bleeding they'd told me about, and corrected that.

Then the orthopedic team took over. The x-rays showed a broken scapula (shoulder blade); several broken ribs; a badly shattered humerus (upper arm bone); broken ulna and radius (lower arm bones); broken hip; and broken femur (thigh bone), tibia, and fibula (lower leg bones)—all down the left side of Larry's body. The humerus and the femur were both compound fractures, meaning the broken edges had torn through muscle and punctured through his skin. They put a rod in the lower leg, a plate in the upper leg, a long screw into the hip, two plates in the lower arm, and two plates in the upper arm. Apparently there was a lot of debris in the mess of his humerus just a few inches above the elbow: glass, pigeon feed from the broken sacks in the trunk, fabric from his shirt, and who knows what else. The doctor was concerned about the severity of that break, and about the rotation of Larry's leg.

It was about 3:30 am when a doctor finally came to take me to the ICU to see Larry after the marathon surgery. He was still sleeping and had been pumped full of fluids, and his face had swollen to the point that I couldn't even see his long eyelashes. Later I read in the records that he'd been given 15 units of blood to replace the many pints he'd lost.

"I've never seen anybody with this many broken bones *live*," the trauma surgeon told me. "He's got some kidney damage, but not from this accident. It's from the years of having diabetes."

I assured the doctor that Larry had a strong will to live and had beaten the odds of medical probabilities before, more than once. He just shook his head.

"We'll see," he said.

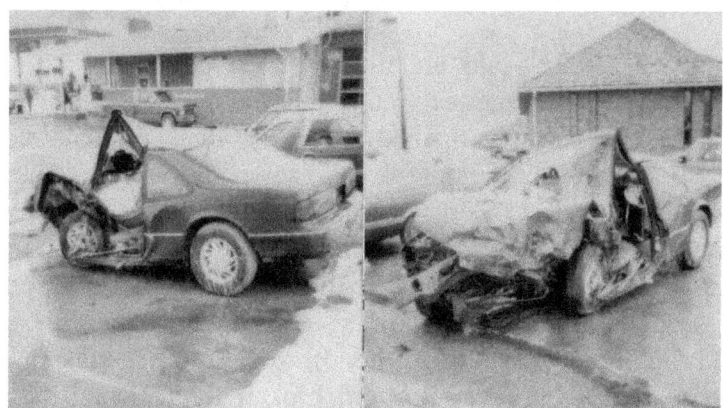

1992 Ford Thunderbird

* * *

Larry stayed in ICU for 1 week, then spent another week and a half on another floor at the hospital before they approved a move to a skilled nursing unit. The cuts on his face were healing, and the stitches were out; ditto the incisions from the surgeries. Now he just needed time to heal and some physical therapy to get his left arm and leg mobile again.

The hospital at Marshall, Missouri, was very new and had a nice skilled nursing unit with only 13 beds, each in individual rooms arranged in a circle around the nurses' station. This meant Larry would have privacy and quiet for sleeping, but plenty of attention from the staff, who were just 10 feet or so away from each of their patients. Marshall was about an hour's drive from our house, but only 30 minutes' drive from my workplace, and being there would get him out of the inner-city environment at Research. After having spent a few days sharing a room with a guy who'd been hit three times in a drive-by shooting (and who then proceeded to conduct his pimping business over the phone from his hospital bed!), Larry was definitely ready to get out of there.

Physical therapy didn't get very far at all before two problems arose: two screws holding the plate on the outer surface of Larry's upper arm broke and the plate bent; then the rod in his lower leg failed because it had been attached by screws near the knee, but not down by the ankle. This did not inspire us to return to Research, so we opted for the orthopedic surgeon on staff at Fitzgibbon, Dr. F. He attached the rod near Larry's ankle and put the leg in a cast for greater stability. Then he replaced the bent plate on the humerus. He removed three of the four broken screw pieces, but was unable to locate one of the screw heads, which had migrated between layers of muscle and never was retrieved for fear that a nerve might be severed while fishing around for it.

Back in the skilled nursing unit, Larry kept a good attitude and followed the guidelines geared toward getting him well. His appetite was good, and they kept a good eye on his blood sugar levels. Whatever they allowed him to do in physical therapy, he was willing to try. The pain of his injuries would never completely go away. With all those metal parts next to his bones, he would learn to dread cold weather. But at the time, these issues hadn't even occurred to us, and he was strictly focused on getting strong enough to come home!

Finally one Thursday his doctor agreed to move him out of skilled nursing and arranged for physical therapy visits at our house. Larry would be coming home, but in a wheelchair—at least for a while.

"Do you have stairs to get into your house?" he asked.

"Yes, there are 4 stairs at the back door and 5 stairs at the front," I confirmed.

"Well, you'll have to make arrangements for a ramp before I can let him leave, then."

I called the house and talked with Mother, who was staying there with Jennifer that week, as she had been doing every other week since the accident. She called Daddy, who hurriedly threw some tools into his station wagon and started driving the 200 miles to our farm, picking up lumber on the way. The two of them and

Jennifer put up a 16-foot ramp with a railing from the lawn to the back door, primed and painted it for protection from the weather, and had it done before I arrived home with Larry the following Saturday afternoon.

It was 7 weeks to the day since the wreck.

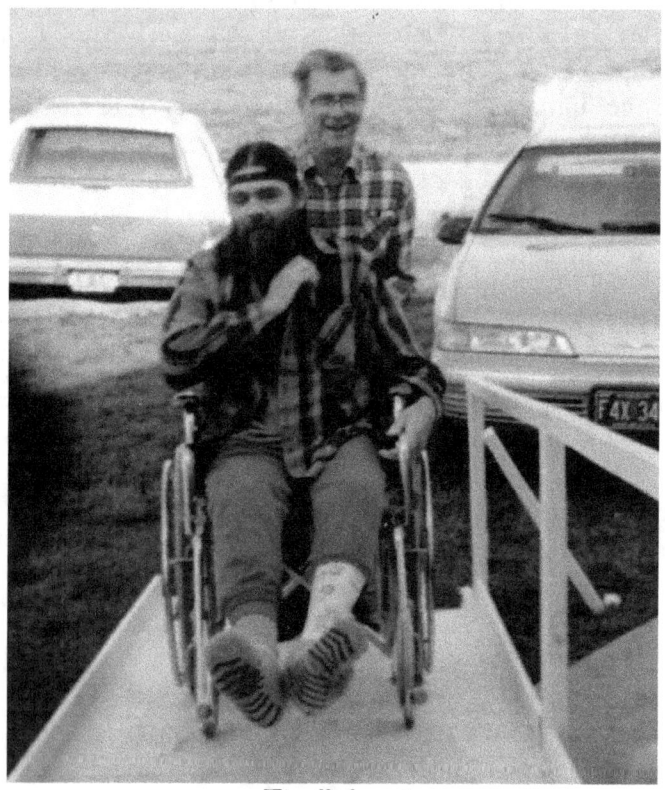

Finally home!

8

SCARY STUFF

Just getting home was a big milestone in Larry's recovery, but the year wasn't over yet... not by a long shot. A visiting nurse came at least three times a week to check his incisions and his blood pressure, look over his blood glucose test results, and watch his overall progress in healing. A physical therapist also began coming in three times a week to work with him on standing and, later, walking with the cast, and in using his left arm. Crutches weren't an option, with his arm having been recently reworked, and within a couple of weeks even the simple exercises of physical therapy caused problems again: screws broke in Larry's upper arm, and the new plate bent. Dr. F. was beside himself, and we weren't too happy either. He wrapped Larry's arm above and below the elbow in a snug bandage and ordered a hinged brace to be worn around the clock.

"If the blood supply to the bone has been too badly compromised, it may not knit back together," he told us. "The bone was badly shattered, and the longer it goes without healing, the lower the chances that it will. You may lose the arm."

We were scared. He told us to give it a few weeks with the brace and then come back for more x-rays, which we did. The cast was removed from Larry's lower leg, as it was healing (although it would always be crooked), but the humerus bone was not making much progress, if any.

Another few weeks with the brace then, and physical therapy at home to help Larry learn to walk again now that the cast was off. This revealed two more problems: his left hip felt "squishy" when he walked, and his left knee and foot angled out to the left instead of straight ahead. When the surgery was done on his femur in Kansas City, it hadn't been aligned properly. So Larry would take a step forward with his artificial right leg, then as he brought his left leg forward, the misaligned foot would swing up and hit the back of his right ankle with the left heel, which risked him tripping and falling with every step. No one wants to fall, but for a guy with this much new metal holding his bones together (well, mostly together), this was truly dangerous.

The surgeon admitted he'd done his best but said it was time to turn the case over to someone who had more expertise than he did with these types of injuries. He told us about Dr. Jeffrey Anglen at University Hospital in Columbia, who'd studied at Johns Hopkins (among other places) and was a specialist in treating patients with mal-unions, non-unions, and polytrauma—in other words, people like Larry! We agreed this sounded like a good plan, and Dr. F. kindly made the arrangements, gave us copies of the x-rays to take with us, and wished us well.

* * *

July 1993

It had been more than 10 years since Larry had been to University Hospital and Clinics in Columbia, Missouri, and what had been a big place was even bigger. We waited anxiously in the orthopedic clinic waiting room, and then in an exam room. Both of us were pretty sure that the loss of an arm would signal the end of Larry's days of riding his precious motorcycle, which was a deprivation too horrible for contemplation, at least to him.

Finally Dr. Anglen came in, greeted us with an easy smile, got a quick summary of the problems, and checked the x-rays.

"Oh, yeah, I can fix that."

He made it sound simple! Dr. Anglen then went on to explain how he would go about the revisions, and looked over his calendar for the first available date. With three separate issues to correct, we knew it would be a lengthy surgery.

Early August arrived, and we made the second of what would prove to be scores of trips to Columbia for medical visits over the coming years. Larry was admitted to the hospital so Dr. Anglen and his team could get to work. It was a long day. First they removed the screws and plate from the back of Larry's femur, cut through the recently-healed bone, rotated the leg back inward so the knee and toes faced forward again, then installed new hardware to hold it there. Secondly the long screw in the hip joint at the top of the femur was removed (there was space between the top of the

60

femur and the knob of bone there, accounting for the "squishy" feeling when walking), matched the two parts back together, and put in an angled metal insert to secure that area. Lastly they drilled out all the screws and removed both plates from the upper arm, slipped in some bone graft material they'd commandeered from Larry's right hip area, and screwed on two new plates, with placement at the back and inside this time, designed to withstand the natural stress that would result during physical therapy. Because they'd cut through the bone at the elbow for access, a small pin was placed there to hold that new separation together, and an anchor wire ran forward from the end of that pin to a tiny angled hole created in the forearm bone, sort of like a guy wire.

Once again, Larry's face and neck were puffy from all the fluids they'd infused during the 6 to 7 hours of surgery. It took a couple of days for the excess liquid to disperse from his system. The morphine they gave him through the IV for pain made him hallucinate and itch, so we asked that they substitute pills instead. He was determined that he would not stay in the hospital a moment longer than necessary, and at the end of the week was thrilled to be released in time to attend our eldest niece's wedding in Springfield. He was in a wheelchair, but he was there!

A month later we returned to Columbia for x-rays to check for progress in the healing of the affected bones. The femur (often a difficult bone to heal, since it is the largest one in the body) was looking great. The hip was intact and knitting well. There was new bone growth showing in the humerus, and the plates were still in place. Finally! The little wire holding the pin in Larry's elbow, however, had slipped out of its mooring, and the pin was starting to back out. Dr. Anglen said this could be a problem and decided to replace the pin with a screw. This was a relatively simple process and was done on an outpatient basis.

Within 10 days the elbow area around the new incision was red, puffy, and warm to the touch; an infection had most likely started when the screw took the place of the pin. Ironic, isn't it, that of all the broken bones they worked on, it was the one they had to cut through that was now causing a challenge? Larry was admitted again and taken back to surgery, where Dr. Anglen and his team cleaned out the infection and packed the tissue with gauze soaked in a special solution to keep the bone, muscle, and skin moist and sterile. Wires were used like twist-ties to keep the incision from gapping any more than was necessary, but not to close it completely; then they wrapped the elbow. A catheter was installed in an artery in Larry's chest for delivery of IV antibiotics. We were sent home with detailed instructions on how to clean and repack the wound to allow it to heal from the inside out. Home health nurses came to our house at 8-hour intervals to infuse the antibiotics and help with wound care. Every few days I used a sterile tool to twist the wires a bit more as the new healthy tissue grew to fill in the gap. We were very grateful the infection had not spread to the bone. Larry stayed on the IV antibiotics for several weeks, then switched to pills. By the time the infection was fully cleared up, the catheter removed, and physical therapy finished, it had been almost a year from the date of his accident.

Dr. Anglen was pleased with the results, but asked us to see him again in a year. "Any time I put this much metal in someone's body, I want to make sure it's holding them together long term," he told us. We saw him annually for the next 5 years before he felt comfortable with a full release.

* * *

Because of the move from Springfield and Larry's lengthy recovery from the accident, we'd had no chance to find a doctor who specialized in regular care of diabetic patients. During Larry's stay in the skilled nursing unit of the hospital at Marshall, he'd been seen by Dr. Koehn, a family practice doctor. They got along well and Larry continued to visit Dr. Koehn every few months afterward for general health maintenance.

One day in late autumn, 1994, Larry seemed to be studying the far side of the room rather intently, shifting his gaze from side to side. He was frowning.

"What's wrong?" I asked.

"I'm not sure," he responded, "but sometimes I'm seeing double."

It was weird. His eyes were tracking together when his gaze was directed straight forward, but when he moved his right eye off to one side or the other, the left eye wasn't following just right; movement was either delayed, or didn't occur at all. By the next morning his left eyelid was starting to droop, and he was feeling some pain at the back of his eye.

Dr. Koehn suspected third nerve palsy, also called cranial mononeuropathy III – diabetic type, or even oculomotor neuropathy. He referred Larry to a neurologist in Columbia, Dr. David McLaren, who confirmed this diagnosis. He explained that this was likely the result of poorly controlled blood sugar levels, that there really wasn't a treatment for it other than trying to keep glucose levels in check, and that it would likely run its course in 3 to 6 months. Usually the muscles that control the eyelid and eye movements return to normal within that period of time. In the meantime, the pain behind Larry's left eye was becoming excruciating to the point of making him nauseous. Strong meds were prescribed for both symptoms, but it was a rough couple of months before he felt like eating much of anything. He had lost a lot of weight after the accident the year before and was just starting to get built back up; this was not a step in the right direction!

Dr. Koehn also told us that while he enjoyed the opportunity to treat Larry, it might be best at this time to transfer his care to another physician he and Dr. McLaren both trusted: Dr. Winkelmeyer, also in Columbia. He made a call and set up an appointment for February.

*   *   *

1995

Dr. Winkelmeyer was a specialist: nephrology and hypertension, the sign said. He dealt with lots of diabetic patients, which naturally included those with kidney problems. He scanned through Larry's lab results.

"In 3 to 5 years—maybe 7—you're going to need dialysis."

We just stared at him. This was our first meeting. How could he predict such a thing? We didn't even think to ask. I almost heard the wheels turning in Larry's mind. *"Not ME!"* he was thinking. I can't recall what I thought exactly, but I do remember the doctor mentioning the possibility of a kidney transplant. It wasn't something we'd ever considered.

So Dr. Winkelmeyer set up a sliding scale for Larry's insulin dosage, recommended he test his blood sugar levels three times a day, and asked us to come see him again in 3 months.

I asked for a copy of the lab report and started a file. Each time Larry saw Dr. W. he received a copy of the lab results, and each page went into the file in chronological order. Usually the blood sugar readings were higher than what the doctor wanted to see. The A1C test is a measure of the blood glucose in one's body over the past 2 to 3 months. Larry's A1C readings were not good. (In February 1995 his A1C was 8.4%; the lab report showed the normal range as 4.3% to 6.1%. His creatinine level was 2.1 mg/dL, which was an indicator of the kidney problems; normal creatinine is 0.6 to 1.2 mg/dL, so Larry's higher level meant his kidneys weren't clearing enough from his system). He dreaded the talks about what typically follows these trends in diabetic patients: hardening of the arteries, heart attack, stroke, kidney failure, vision loss, nephropathy, circulation problems... call it the Ostrich Syndrome, denial, or whatever. His rebel nature didn't want to believe those things could happen to him.

But as a wife and a helpmate, I could not put my head in the sand and pretend the threat would just go away. My reminders to "do your test" before meals and bedtime weren't always well received, but were honored. Dr. W. wanted to see those test sheets at each appointment and would sometimes circle the readings that were dangerously higher than Larry's recommended target of 150. "Over 500" was the highest possible reading on the meter, and there were often several such readings in a 3-month batch of test sheets. The lab reports might have the BUN (blood urea nitrogen) and creatinine figures circled, both of which are measures of kidney function. Dr. Winkelmeyer was doing his best to help preserve Larry's health as long as possible.

Our daughter Jennifer wasn't exempt from the effects of Larry's illness. Once, as a young girl, she had realized Larry was going into an insulin reaction, and raided her own Easter basket to bring him something she knew would help bring his blood sugar up to an acceptable level. But probably the worst incident she ever experienced occurred when she was in high school, shortly after Larry got his first insulin pump.

When we were trained by a nurse-educator in how to set up and use the insulin pump, she provided a prescription for an emergency Glucagon kit, and encouraged us to fill it immediately. At the time, we had no prescription insurance that covered Larry, and the kit cost $98.00, but we spent the money and stashed the kit in the bathroom cabinet.

About 2 weeks later, Larry went into another insulin reaction, and this one hit him hard and fast. In spite of Jennifer's best efforts with the normal antidotes of food and drink, her dad seemed to keep slipping further and further away. I was out on a job, but she reached me by cell phone, and I told her to get the little red kit from the medicine cabinet and give an emergency injection of Glucagon to her dad. Thank God her boyfriend (and future husband) BJ was near enough to race over and administer the shot, because in her panic and fear of hurting him, Jennifer was simply not able to get that needle into the muscle of Larry's upper arm. And let me tell you: if you've never had to give anyone a shot of anything, it's much harder than you think. Those little syringe needles are sharp, but the skin of an arm can be tough. How in the world Larry ever learned to give himself insulin at the age of 7 is still beyond me.

It took several tense minutes for the Glucagon to hit Larry's bloodstream and bring him around, but it worked. Jennifer made her dad a couple of sandwiches, then, and brought them to him with a large glass of milk. They all breathed a huge sigh of relief. Larry told Jennifer and BJ that he had felt like he was "leaving", and he was scared. Jennifer replied that she was scared, too! And as soon as I arrived home and heard all about the incident, I determined that we'd be getting a replacement Glucagon kit for the medicine cabinet immediately. It was most definitely worth the cost.

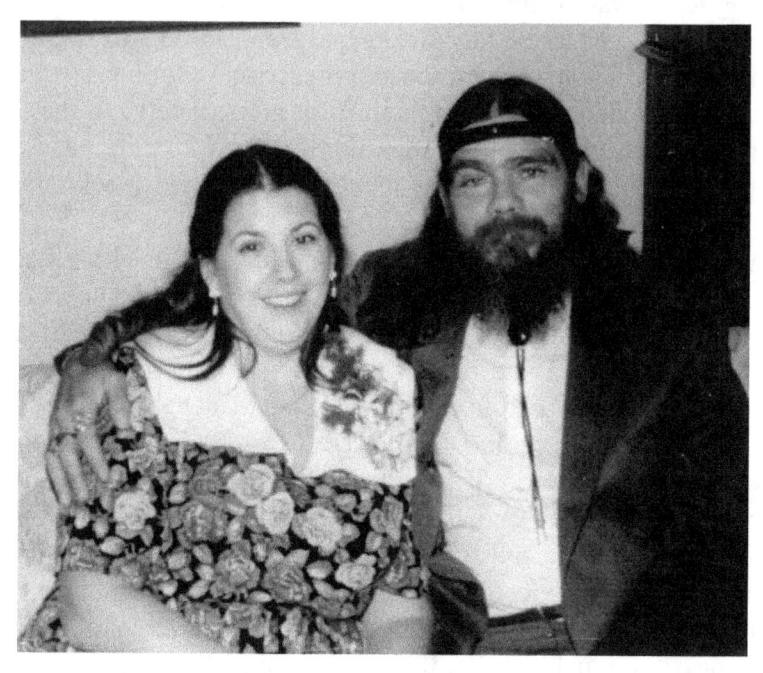

Jesse and Larry, 1995 (photo credit Alma Weilmuenster)

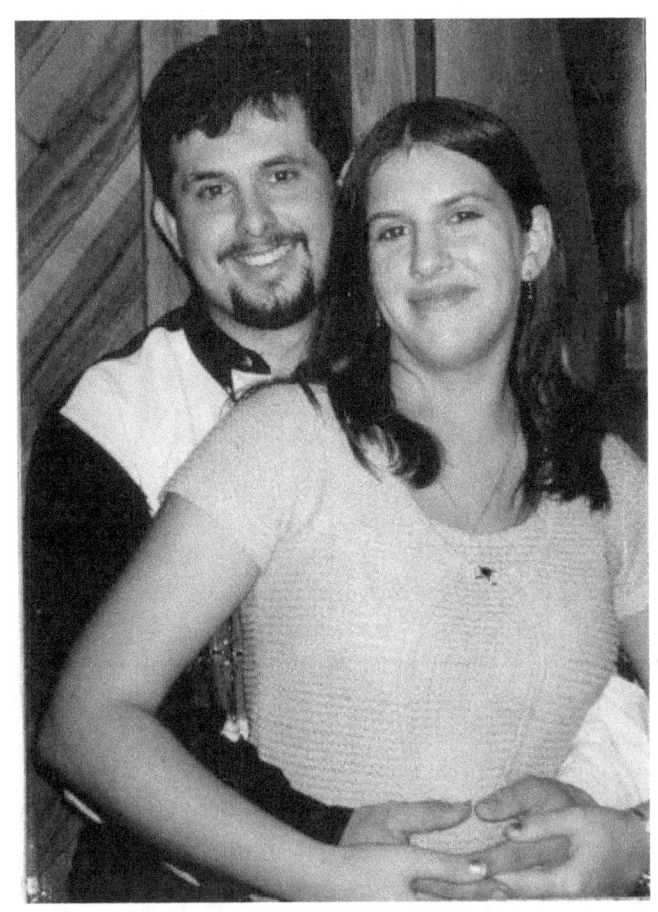

BJ and Jennifer

9
MATTERS OF THE HEART

July, 1998

Just before the 4th of July, on a Friday morning, Larry didn't feel well. He had an upset stomach first of all. Thinking it was acid indigestion, he asked for Alka-Seltzer. Mindful of the salt content of that product, and his compromised kidneys, I suggested Tums instead. Those didn't help. Larry was still in bed when I was talking on the phone with my sister Janice, who lives in Texas. At her question on exactly how he was feeling, he said "Like there's a concrete block sitting on my chest."

"Oh, my," Janice spoke cautiously, "he needs to be checked out. That could be a heart attack symptom."

I called the local family doctor who I saw for occasional minor issues, and the receptionist said we could come right in as soon as possible. Larry protested a little but still wasn't feeling better, so got up and dressed to go. The doctor listened to Larry's heart and lungs and said he didn't think it was anything much to be concerned about, but that it might not be a bad idea to drive up to Sedalia and have the ER team at the hospital there run an electrocardiogram (EKG).

So off we went. It was just a 30-minute drive, and the ER team got right to work. They drew blood, ran the EKG, and gave Larry a liquid antacid that seemed to give him almost immediate relief. "OK!" we thought. "That's a good sign."

Jennifer and I were in the waiting room when a young doctor came out to discuss the situation. He looked a little stunned, and told us that in spite of the help the antacid had provided, the blood test didn't lie… Larry had suffered a heart attack. "A mild one," he told us. "We'd like to keep him here for observation over the weekend. He'll be in the Cardiac Care Unit, on a monitor, so if his heart starts acting up again we'll know it instantly. On Monday we can transfer him by ambulance over to one of the hospitals in

Columbia for more tests."

"What sort of tests?" I asked. "And can they not be done here?"

"Well, they'll probably start with a stress test. If that indicates an irregularity, he may need an angiogram or even surgery; it's safer for Larry if he's already there where they can perform those procedures. We have the capability to do the test, but it can sometimes trigger another heart attack. In someone who has just *had* one, we prefer to get them to the larger facility before risking that. And with the holiday weekend starting... it'll be Monday before we can move him there."

"But what if he goes into distress again over the weekend, here?" I queried.

"Then his condition would go from stable to serious or critical, and we'd get him into the helicopter immediately," the doctor reassured me. "They do take new cases over the weekend on an emergency basis. Right now, however, Larry's condition doesn't warrant that."

So Larry was made as comfortable as possible in the CICU, hooked up to monitors, and told he had to stay in bed. A trip to the bathroom required nursing assistance. He felt caged. He got bored. He watched the lines on the cardiac monitor, separate readings for pulse, blood pressure, respirations, oxygen saturation. Hmm... what would happen if he breathed fast, as if he was panting... Ooh! Lots of squiggles on the screen. Then another experiment: he held his breath. A couple of the lines went still, although obviously, not the one for heart rate. All the same, the alarms started chiming and in ran the nurse, only to see Larry reclined (almost sitting) in the bed, smiling like an angel. Well, OK... a mischievous angel.

"Don't you *ever* do that again!" she admonished him. He kept smiling, a twinkle in his eyes, but minded his manners after that.

On Monday Larry was transported to Boone Hospital in Columbia as planned and met Dr. Tony Spaedy, a cardiologist we soon came to trust and respect. He found one blocked artery and put in a stent (an expandable metal mesh tube) to help hold it open. He told us the artery had been 95% blocked, and the blockage was the cause of Larry's heart attack. The other arteries around his

69

heart were 30% to 35% blocked, but for now did not need intervention. He prescribed Lipitor for cholesterol control, and atenolol, a pill that can help prevent second heart attacks. It can also treat high blood pressure.

Dr. Spaedy's office was in the building next door to Dr. Winkelmeyer's, and the two doctors already knew each other and worked well together. When he found out that Larry was already on a schedule of quarterly visits with Dr. Winkelmeyer, Dr. Spaedy told us Larry was in good hands. He knew he'd be called if there was a problem.

*   *   *

February, 2000

The stent opened up that artery to vastly improve the blood flow to Larry's heart and helped him feel better for well over a year. The long-term effects of diabetes, however, were continually working, and not in Larry's favor. By the winter of 1999–2000, he was getting lethargic, and seemed to get out of breath more easily. Some days, just walking 120 feet or so down the driveway to the mailbox was taxing to his system.

"Do you think it's your heart?" I asked, half-afraid of what the answer might be, but needing to know nonetheless.

"Yeah, maybe," Larry admitted.

"Might be a good idea to call Dr. Spaedy, have it checked out," I ventured, thinking this suggestion would likely be met with resistance. But he surprised me this time.

"Oh, I guess so. Probably ought to," was the response.

Wow. For Larry to admit this meant that he must be feeling even worse than I knew! He dealt with a lot of pain every day, including arthritis from the injuries of the past, but this category of pain was apparently different, and bothered him enough to agree to seek help.

So I made the call, and Dr. Spaedy's nurse set up an appointment, which led to tests, which led to an admission to Boone Hospital. This time there were four or five blockages, and it was time for bypass surgery. Larry was 50 years old, and less than thrilled with the prospect. In fact, he was being downright stubborn about it. He wanted out of there, wanted to go home.

Dr. Spaedy talked to him about the operation, and why he felt this was truly a necessary procedure.

Dr. Winkelmeyer came in an hour later and offered his opinion on how this option could extend Larry's life, hopefully by many years.

Larry's brother Tom talked with him, too, trying to provide reassurance that God can work through doctors, and that He does so every day, in many ways.

I reminded my husband that we had a teenaged daughter at home and that she and I both still needed and wanted him around!

Finally, Larry relented and agreed to the surgery, which resulted in five bypasses of the arteries around his heart. He weathered it well, and they had him up and moving around (with a walker and help, of course) within a day. After a relatively normal recovery, he completed the cardiac rehabilitation program at Bothwell Hospital in Sedalia, since it was much closer to home than Boone. Once again, he amazed the therapists in the clinic with his positive attitude and his tenacity to go the distance, meeting and often exceeding the goals they set for him in each phase of exercise.

With a warning against extreme exertion and advice not to spend more than 15 to 20 minutes outside during very hot or very cold weather, Larry was released from care by the surgeon and by Dr. Spaedy.

"Call me if you need me," Dr. S. said with a smile.

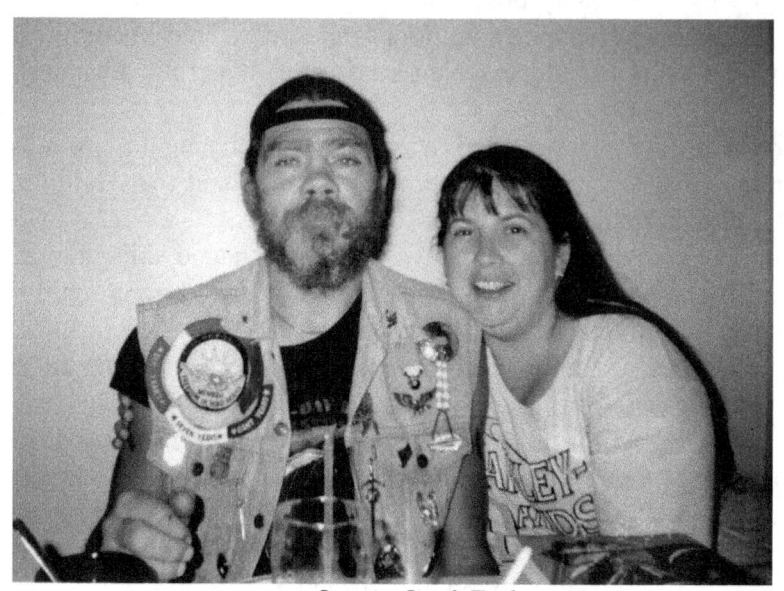

Sturgis, South Dakota

10
PAPA AND GRANDPA

The next decade seemed to pass as a blur of activity.

2001 was notable for that terrible event that affected all Americans in one way or another—the attacks on the Twin Towers and the Pentagon, and the fourth plane that went down in Pennsylvania—which happened to coincide with my 40th birthday. Like so many other folks, we spent a good part of the day in front of the television, struggling to comprehend what was happening and why.

2002 saw celebrations for our daughter Jennifer's marriage to BJ Martinez and later the birth of our first grandchild, Lily. There's something indescribably special about holding the child of your child, and we both instantly adored this precious bundle. Papa Larry had the honor—and the responsibility—of staying with Lily every morning while Jennifer was taking classes, forming an extremely close bond between the bearded biker and the happy baby.

2003 marked Jennifer's graduation with honors from high school, and the beginning of her classes at State Fair Community College in Sedalia.

2004 began with the arrival of our only grandson, Luke. Jennifer returned to classes within a week of his arrival, BJ started working nights, and they all four moved into the farmhouse with us for a good part of the year. Papa didn't have to go anywhere to help with the little ones, Jennifer and the children weren't alone at night, and BJ worked hard to save money for a down payment on a house of their own. Their first night in their new home was Christmas Eve. Meanwhile, mid-year, my parents celebrated their 50th wedding anniversary!

In the midst of all the activity, however, Larry's beloved mama was dying. She'd successfully fought breast cancer several years before, but this time was different. PET scans showed cancer now growing in both lungs. She and John were in health care facilities in Springfield, and Larry tried to make the 2-hour drive to see them as often as possible. With his commitment to babysitting Lily and Luke, this didn't happen as often as he liked, but he did his best. In July 2004 Nadine succumbed to the cancer, slipping away quietly in the night. Susan, Larry, and Tom met later in the morning to make the arrangements for her service.

Jennifer, Lily, and Luke went with Larry and me to the funeral in Springfield. Luke, just 6 months old, spent most of his time on his mama's lap. Lily, a month away from turning 2 years old, took turns between Larry's lap, mine, and cousin Dana, who'd made the trip from Colorado for the service. We were a somber bunch, and it wasn't a situation Lily had experienced before; it didn't take long for her to notice the difference. Her Papa wasn't teasing, laughing, or grinning at her. In fact, as she gazed up into his sad face, two fat tears were rolling down his cheeks.

"Papa, wha's matter?" Lily asked softly, an expression of deep concern on her tiny face.

Larry looked down and patted her back. "It's OK, honey. Papa's alright."

"'S'matter, Papa?" she quizzed again, more insistent this time. She knew better than to believe the first version, not with evidence otherwise running down her precious Papa's face.

"It's OK" he whispered again, "I'm just sad today. I'll be OK though."

Lily was thoughtful, wishing she knew how to help Papa, as he always seemed to help her.

"Got Neenex?" she asked.

Larry shook his head in the negative. I leaned over and whispered in his ear that he'd find a clean handkerchief in the inside chest pocket of his suit coat. He reached in and retrieved it. Lily immediately took it from him and gently dabbed at his tears, smiling at him in encouragement.

It was a moment of such compassion from Miss Lily. Her gentle act of kindness was indelibly etched in our list of favorite memories as grandparents, in spite of the reason for the event.

2005 was the year Larry's back started really bothering him a lot. He tried chiropractic care, then epidural injections, and later physical therapy. The diagnosis was "degenerative disk disease," which may have been hereditary, as he recalled his maternal granddad had had the same symptoms. Larry had lost a little height after all the leg surgeries following his car accident in 1993, but now seemed to start shrinking in stature a bit more.

May 2006 should have found Jennifer in a cap and gown again, receiving her Associate's Degree, except that she was in the hospital in Clinton that day, giving birth to her second daughter, Megan. This sweet little girl loves to snuggle, but in spite of her tiny frame, has spunk and a fierce protectiveness of her siblings that gets a nod of respect from all of us… and sometimes a laugh as well.

Also in 2006, around the time of his birthday, Larry was coming up the back steps to the house when the locking pin mechanism that held his prosthetic leg in place (the designs had changed over the years) failed, the leg came loose, and Larry fell off the side of the steps, breaking one of the bones in his left forearm just behind the plate that had been in place since 1993. A local doctor splinted and wrapped it. A few days later Dr. Todd Oliver, an orthopedic surgeon in Columbia, provided a brace.

2007 arrived a few months later, but still the fractured arm wasn't healing. Dr. Oliver arranged for Larry to get an electronic bone growth stimulation device, which he used at home daily for months. Some progress resulted, but "nothing to write home about," as my mother would say. Dr. O diagnosed this as a hypertrophic non-union, and performed surgery on November 28, removing the old plate, adding some allograft putty and chips of bone from the new growth where his body had tried to heal the fracture, and centering a new plate over the area.

A couple of weeks prior to that surgery, Larry and I took our grandson Luke to Sedalia one evening. Luke (or "Bubba" as we often call him) was, at that time, a couple of months away from turning 4 years old. At the movie theater we saw "Bee Movie," a really cute animated film. To top off the thrill, we made a stop at Baskin-Robbins ice cream shop. Luke had never seen so many choices! After enjoying the treat it was time to head for home.

With Larry driving and Luke in his car seat behind me, we took the backroads west, then south of town toward the farm. The moon was full and bright in the west, shining over the dormant farmlands in a brilliant glow.

"Bubba, look!" I exclaimed, "Look out your window… do you see that big ol' moon up there?"

"Yes!" he confirmed, then: "God live inna moon."

"What's that?"

He repeated the statement.

"God lives in the moon?" I asked him.

"Yes," Bubba told me, very confidently.

"Uh, well… I thought God lives in Heaven," was my reply.

"Uh-huh," he agreed. "God live in Heaven, 'n Heaven is inna guy [sky], anna moon is inna guy, so God live in Heaven inna moon inna guy."

Oh my. What fine reasoning! For someone almost 4 years old, this deduction made perfect sense, and Luke presented it with great aplomb. How could a grandma argue with that?

"OK, Bubba, that sounds good to me."

"Uh-huh," he continued calmly "and someday, when we die and the angels come and snatch us from our beds, we go live with God in Heaven inna moon inna guy."

I took a moment to digest that one. The mental image of angels snatching us from our beds was really something to ponder.

"Well, yes, honey, I believe we will," I ventured, "but not right now."

"No, not now," he concurred. "Someday."

"That's right," Larry finally joined in. "Someday."

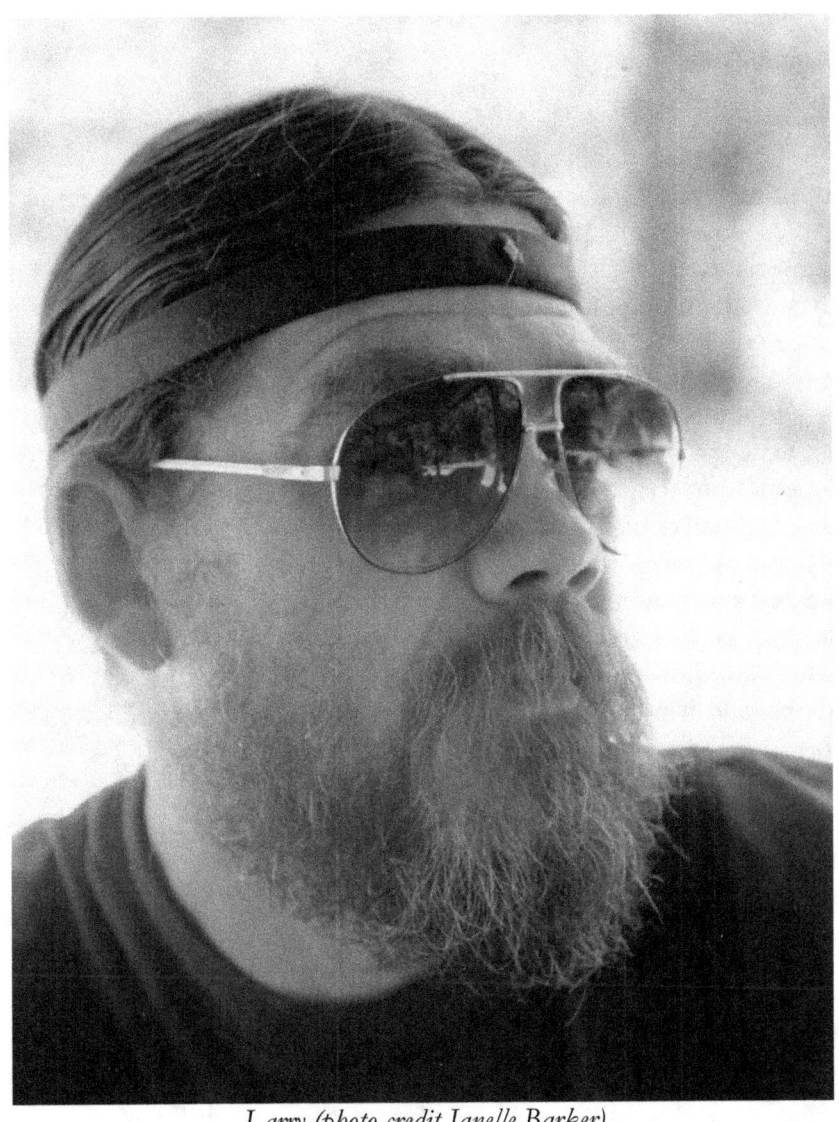

Larry (photo credit Janelle Barker)

11
ESRD

The winter months had become harder for Larry each year, especially after the bypass surgery, and included almost annual battles with bronchitis. February to March of this year saw the same pattern: What started as a head cold quickly went into his chest with bronchitis and then to pneumonia, even though he'd received a pneumonia vaccine the preceding November. After a few days in the hospital in early March, Dr. Winkelmeyer prescribed antibiotics and breathing treatments using a nebulizer at home. The illness started to clear up, but Larry was weak, had little appetite, and felt draggy all the time. His cough just wouldn't go away. Finally, at the beginning of April when I called Dr. W's office and spoke with Anita Cox, the nurse practitioner, she broke the news as gently as possible: More antibiotics probably wouldn't do the trick. Larry needed to go on dialysis. His kidneys had deteriorated to the point that his body was carrying too many toxins, and it was affecting his ability to fight off infections of this sort.

I told Larry what she'd said and he shook his head "no." She advised me to talk it over with him and let her know the decision as soon as possible. Anita had been Dr. W's nurse when we first started going to that office, and had been a reliable care partner for years. I knew she was only telling me what we needed to hear.

It was morning and Larry was still in bed. I sat down at the foot of the bed and we talked about it. For years, his mantra regarding dialysis had been "it's never going to happen." He'd long held the opinion that we shouldn't "curse" ourselves by giving voice to negative possibilities, even if they were probabilities or what medical professionals called "eventualities." Our faith in God and His ability to heal physical ailments was strong and unshakable. Maybe Larry felt like admitting it was time for dialysis was akin to doubting God? I asked him about that.

He nodded. I tried to reassure him.

"Honey, it's not making a statement that you don't believe God can heal… it's recognizing that God works through doctors and nurses and medical devices, too. What they're telling us is that if you don't do dialysis, you won't get better. That would be giving up! Since when are you a quitter?!"

"I'm not," he replied.

"And I'm not ready to lose you," I said.

Our gazes held. I offered a small questioning smile. Larry drew as deep a breath as possible and let it out slowly. We both cried a little.

"OK," he finally said quietly, "I'll do it."

* * *

Within a couple of hours we were on the way to Columbia for what would soon become scores of regular trips to that town. Larry's attitude was positive now, almost a complete reversal of his earlier tone. I complimented him on this.

"I just had to get my head around it," he said.

Once he made up his mind about something, there wasn't much that could hold him back from making it work.

Dr. Winkelmeyer met us at Boone Hospital, where Larry was admitted for his first dialysis treatment on April 2, 2008. My parents met us there and kept us company for a while, marveling at Larry's smiles and offering words of encouragement to us both.

The next day Larry had outpatient surgery to install a Permacath, which allows ready access to a large central vein in the chest for dialysis. The access ports were on the ends of two small plastic tubes that exited his chest a few inches right of center. The exit site had to be kept dry at all times, and carefully cleaned daily to prevent infection. About a week later the vascular surgeon also moved a vein in Larry's left arm to create an arteriovenous (AV) fistula, which would be used instead of the Permacath once the fistula "matured." This vein eventually would become large and ropey looking under the surface of his skin, and we could begin to feel a "buzz" in it as it grew over the following months.

79

Dialysis clinics have become commonplace in cities and are being built in more moderate-sized towns all the time; there were already units in Sedalia and Clinton, each within an easy 30-minute drive of our home. But to receive dialysis service at either of these clinics, Larry would have needed to be under the care of a local doctor associated with one of them. After working with Dr. Winkelmeyer for more than 12 years, we really didn't want to jump ship now. So Larry made the 180-mile roundtrip drive to and from Columbia 3 days a week for the next several weeks.

Dr. W. had told us about a rather new method of receiving dialysis at home, through a company called NxStage®. Although it was not uncommon for patients to perform peritoneal dialysis at home in 2008, hemodialysis outside of a hospital or clinic was a relatively rare occurrence at that time. Lisa Baker, the facilitator of the DaVita dialysis clinic in Columbia, talked to Larry about the program and came to visit our home. She looked over the storage area I'd cleared in the library closet and recommended I make more room on the shelves for supplies. She described the 3-week training program Larry would need to complete before they'd bring the machine to the house, and asked if I'd be able to attend with him.

"Five days a week, for 3 straight weeks?" I repeated. "In the middle of May?" I tried to explain that my job as a property claims adjuster meant long hours during the spring and summer storm season, and that while I did get a certain number of vacation days each year, those were generally prescheduled for the year back in January, with supervisors trying to juggle the delicate balance between having enough personnel to provide prompt service to our customers while still accommodating the needs of the employees.

"I'll see what I can do," I told her, "but 1 week is probably the most I can hope for at this time of year."

"Make it the last week, then," Lisa told me. "By then he should have the routine under his belt, and you can learn from him how to be 'back-up' in case he needs your help."

She had one more question for me.

"Do you think he can do this?"

There was no doubt in my mind. "Oh, yes," I told her. "If Larry is determined to make something work, he can—and will—definitely do it!"

* * *

Instead of being hooked up to one of the regular dialyzers in the big room of the clinic on Monday, May 11, Larry met with Nurse Lisa in a smaller training room across from her office, and began learning about the NxStage System One cycler and the PureFlow dialysate cabinet and control unit.

Peritoneal dialysis uses osmosis to draw toxins from the patient's body by infusing dialysate directly into the abdominal cavity through a catheter, allowing it to "dwell" there a few hours, and then draining it away. Contrary to this, during hemodialysis the patient's blood is drawn out of his or her body through tubing (the Arterial line), channeled through the semi-permeable membrane of a filter, and then returned to the patient via another tube called the Venous line. The filter itself is in a sturdy plastic cartridge and is surrounded by dialysate fluid, which is continuously moving in the opposite direction from the blood before going down a drain, taking waste products, such as urea, and excess fluids with it. Nurse Lisa calls this tube the "pee line."

Apparently a good percentage of folks who need dialysis have kidneys that have shut down so entirely that they no longer pee at all. Every doctor or nurse visit from this point forward, they'd ask Larry if he still made urine. He'd assure them he did.

"How much?" was the next question.

"How the hell should I know?!" was the answer he wanted to give, but didn't. "I don't measure it," was the usual answer; "Some days more than others" or "Two to three times a day" were alternatives. Geez! If they actually expected him to measure the stuff, why did they never say so? (Conversely, if you were a medical professional and always had to ask the question, you might think that repeated monthly visits with the same list of questions might lead someone to realize that maybe they should start measuring...)

After the first week of dialysis, however, we could tell that it was definitely helping to remove some bad stuff, because Larry felt so much better! He was able to attend his dad's 80th birthday party in Springfield that weekend, and he had a good appetite for the special dinner that was planned.

On May 8 he saw Dr. Oliver for a check-up on the left forearm fracture, and finally got a hopeful prognosis.

"There's quite a bit of new bone growth there," the doctor told us. "It's looking considerably better than it has before."

We explained that Larry had begun dialysis just about 5 weeks previous.

"Ah," he nodded. "I figured that was what it would take." He went on to explain that kidney failure inhibits the body's production of red blood cells, and that the ones it does make don't live as long, thereby restricting one's ability to heal in many ways.

Future follow-up visits in July and September confirmed the continued successful healing of the bone.

But to get back to the training... Larry had daily treatments 5 days a week for 2 weeks with the new equipment and Nurse Lisa's teaching, along with large binders and spiral notebooks to study afterward. The third week I went with him. Lisa explained that hooking up the tubes seemed to be giving my husband a little trouble due to the arthritis in his hands and the steadiness and fine motor skills required for some of the tiny caps and connectors. We worked out a routine that split the required preparations into things that he could do and things that I'd do for him. She had a list of steps printed out on paper and taped to the wall by the recliner where he sat. During training, we made a few adjustments and additions to the list before printing out a new copy that we brought home. I was glad to be able to confirm that we'd completed the list of preparatory steps at home:

- Two GFCI (ground fault circuit interrupter) outlets had been installed in the living room, one on each side of the room in the areas where Larry might want to sit during his treatment.

- A phone jack with a line splitter was added to the living room, for occasional online updates between NxStage and their machine.

- A small sink and vanity were put in the dining room (our living/dining areas are one long room), within several feet of Larry's favorite spot on the reclining end of the sofa. This supplied clean cold water for the PureFlow unit to mix with the bags of dialysate concentrate in the cabinet unit, and also a drain line for it to exit after use.

- A total of 300 cubic feet of closet area was cleared and made ready for boxes of supplies. (This proved to be a bit insufficient and the closet too far away, and eventually a lot of the stuff sort of "migrated" and took over our dining room).

- The electric cooperative office was notified that we'd be doing dialysis treatments at home, and they put us on the "priority list" for repair service in the event of a power outage.

On the last Friday in May, Nurse Lisa came to the house with another RN, Karen Jacobi, who was going to be working with home hemo patients as well. The UPS driver had been busy delivering boxes of supplies over the previous couple of weeks, and with the NxStage cycler now in place, we were ready to get started. We'd had a "dress rehearsal" at the DaVita clinic the day before, when Larry and I executed all the steps to set up, perform, and complete the treatment, while Lisa observed and made herself available for questions or possible complications. It had gone well, and this first treatment at home would prove the same. Both nurses were there for observation and any needed assistance, and both of their names and phone numbers were posted on the front of the machine for future reference. Thank you, ladies! They had to answer a *lot* of questions over the next few years, and especially during the first months.

The dialysis machine and all the accompanying supplies took up a good bit of space, and the treatments seemed to take over a large portion of our lives. Beforehand, we'd heard "2 to 3 hours a day"; in actuality, we spent about 4 to 5 hours a day the first several months, because the speed of the cycler must be kept lower when using the Permacath. In October 2008, Larry's AV fistula (that big ropey vein with the funny buzzing feel in his left upper arm above the elbow) was ready to use, and over time we were able to increase the speed of the cycler by increments. The length of treatments also depended in part on how much extra fluid we had to draw off each day. The nurses had brought a digital scale to the house that took readings in pounds or kilograms, and for some reason, medical things are all factored in kilos. Larry stepped on the scale for a reading before and after treatment, and these were recorded on a chart along with blood pressure, pulse, and a lot of other variables every time. The chart, called a flow sheet, was to be faxed in to our dialysis nurse within 30 minutes of the completion of treatment, without fail.

Lisa warned us, "If I don't get your flow sheet, I will be calling you. And if you fail to send in 3 sheets in a row, I'll be there to pick up the machine."

This was not a warning we took lightly, and we were diligent about sending the sheets. We knew Lisa was accountable to DaVita and to Dr. Winkelmeyer, to verify that Larry was receiving the care he needed, and therefore we were accountable to her, and later to Nurse Karen. Medicare and Larry's supplemental insurance were paying for the service, and could demand proof of it at any time, too. The paperwork had to be there.

For the curious, the nearby figure shows what Larry's flow sheet looked like at the time.

Home at HOME

Fax Completed Treatment Sheet to your clinic # __1889__ _____ **at End of Treatment**

NxStage Hemo Dialysis Flowsheet

PATIENT NAME: ____ Larry Crain

Date: _____

Bar Code #: _____

Flowsheet ID #: _____

Nephrologist _____

Reviewed by RN _____ Dr. Winkelmyer

PRE-TREATMENT VITALS

Sitting BP	Pulse
Stand BP	Pulse
Temp °F	
Previous Post Weight	
Today's Weight	
Dry Weight (-)	66
Fluid to Remove (=)	

Lab Tubes Drawn

SST	Dark Blue
Green	Light Blue
Lavender	Other

Dialysate / Product Water Testing

	Product Water (if applicable)
Dialysate	
Culture	Culture
LAL	LAL

PRE-TREATMENT DATA COLLECTION

Day of the Week Mon Tue Wed Th Fr Sat Sun

Short of Breath	Y N	Change in Mobility	Y N
Swelling	Y N	Digestion Problems	Y N
Hosp/ER/Procedure/accident/fall since last treatment? Y N (If yes, Call HHD)		Access(es) in Place Fistula/Graft/Catheter	
Nurse before Starting Treatment)		Access(es) in Use Fistula/Graft/Catheter	
Access - any redness/drainage/swelling? Y N (If yes, Call HHD Nurse before Starting Treatment)		If Fistula/Graft, Thrill&Bruit? Y N	
		If Catheter, Dressing Changed Y N	
		Catheter function: good poor	

Dialysis Orders

Volume 25L		Filtration Fraction	30
Lactate	40 K+	Access AVF	Loc Lft Upper
Sak# 001 002 003 004 005	1K	Needle Gau	15 Length 1in
Blood Flow Rate	550	Heparin (1000 units/ml)	.000

Drugs Administered

Heparin Bolus (1000 units/ml)		Dose 6000 /IVP	Route Time Initial
EPO			

Notes: _____

Time	BP	Pulse	Dialysate (Green) Rate Volume	UF (Yellow) Rate Volume	Blood Flow Rate(Rad)	Arterial Pressure	Venous Pressure	Effluent Pressure	Access	Saline	Remarks	Initials

Start Time _____ Stop Time _____

POST-TREATMENT DATA COLLECTION

Short of Breath Y N	If Fistula/Graft,Thrill&Bruit? Y N	Bruising Y N	
Swelling Y N	Bleeding Stop Time ___ min.	Infiltration Y N	
Digestion Problems Y N			

Post Treatment Vital Signs

Sitting BP	Pulse
Standing BP	Pulse
Temp °F	Post Weight
Total Time:	Total Dialysate:
Missed Treatment due to (circle one):	

Total UF: _____ Total BVP: _____ Dialyzer Post: (circle one) Clear Streaked Clotted

Other/Explain: _____

Lot Numbers

Cartridge Lot #	
SAK Lot #	
Cycler #	7108
Warmer Serial #	C101159
Control Panel Serial #	D6130

Machine Checks

Alarm Test Completed:	Y N
Total Chlorine Check	
SAK Test# 1 2 3 Bag Y N	
Total Chlorine Level <0.1ppm >0.1ppm	

Signatures: _____

85

Once a month we drew lab samples. The clinic provided the variety of test tubes needed and showed us (and provided a chart in the learning materials for reference) how the different colored stoppers in the tops represented separate protocols. The red stopper with black marbling in it had a gel material in the bottom. After filling it via a Vacutainer plugged in to the arterial line, it had to sit upright 30 minutes before being spun in a centrifuge, after which the blood solids would be on the bottom, the gel in the middle, and the almost-clear plasma on the top. Then it went into the refrigerator. Little foam blocks with holes in them were provided to hold the tubes upright and cushioned for safety. Lavender-topped tubes were smaller, but we usually drew 3 or 4 of those. They went directly into refrigeration. After treatment there was a marbled green/black-topped tube—again with gel—that didn't have to wait to go into the centrifuge. Plus, there was either a large tube (or later a special bag with a sealable connector) for a sample of the dialysate from the machine. All of these containers were labeled with Larry's name, a bar code, and the date.

Since Larry's weekday treatments were conducted in the evening after my workday, the samples were shipped the next morning. I would call FedEx the night before to schedule a pickup, and the usual driver who came from Sedalia was about as regular as clockwork. I knew to be watching for Matt about 9:35 am, and would have the box ready to go. The samples were loaded into a sealable plastic bag with a sheet of absorbent fabric "just in case." Into the box was placed a cushioned liner that helped hold the temperature within, then a frozen cold-pack was put inside with paper towels on top, followed by the sealed bag of samples. The liner was folded shut, the lab requisition forms added on top, and the box sealed. A pre-printed label was attached called a "prepaid billable stamp" for next-day delivery, so we didn't have to pay the pickup driver or take the box to a FedEx center. The clinic had obviously put some thought into this entire process, and had a chart printed up in our reference book showing all the steps for this monthly routine also. They even supplied the strip of clear plastic tape to secure the lid of the box!

Generally "lab days" were Wednesdays, and Larry's nurse

would often get the results the following Monday. She would note any irregularities and send the report on to Dr. Winkelmeyer with her suggestions (if any) for adjustments in medications or treatment protocol. Within a week after this, one day was usually the appointed monthly clinic visit, when Larry would meet with Dr. W, his dialysis nurse (Lisa, then Karen, or later, Allie for several months), a dietician (Suzette), and a social worker (Sarah). Larry would be given a copy of the lab results, and any anomalies would be discussed. I soon asked that the nurse fax or email a copy of the lab report to me when she received it, so that I could watch the trends in Larry's numbers and talk with him about them, enabling us to formulate our questions before the clinic meetings, which seemed to go by way too quickly for us. I kept these reports in the file with the others from his blood work over the years, with the newest ones placed in the back each time. This made it easy to locate and review his lab results from any given date over the past several years.

12
BOXES AND MORE BOXES

One of the surprising things about conducting Larry's dialysis treatments at home was the amount of space required for the necessary supplies and the number of hours I spent keeping track of it all. Two separate inventories had to be completed each month by particular dates.

The NxStage customer service department provided a one-page inventory form that listed Larry's name and patient number. I filled in the serial numbers from their cycler and from the control panel for the PureFlow unit. The PureFlow required a large heavy filter box called a PurePak to remove any possible sediment and impurities from our household water before mixing it with the dialysate concentrate to make a 60-liter "batch." Our farm has a deep well with what I consider good water, but it is "hard" water with substantial mineral content such as lime and calcium. We discovered a PurePak would last only about 3 weeks at our place; for a patient who lives in town with a city water source, it might last 3 months. Supplies were delivered to us monthly by UPS, so I figured we should always have two extra PurePaks on hand. Initially it sounded like one stand-by should be enough. When the filter had been used as long as it should, the warning light and display readout on the PureFlow would advise me it was time to prime a new one. I'd remove the used one (at that point it's really heavy!); install the new box; hook up the computer plug-in, the water supply, and the connector tube to the control module; and push the button for it to prime. This process took about 2½ hours. At the end of that time the control unit would beep again to indicate that it was done, and the display would tell me to close the clamps on the connector line. Then I could either shut down the machine for the night and make myself a note to start making a new batch of dialysate in the morning, or else proceed with loading a "sak" (the NxStage term for the heavy plastic bag with the dialysate concentrate) for the following day's treatment. Just a couple of months into the process, however, when the machine had primed a new Pak, instead of having "prime complete, close clamps" on the readout, it said something like "conductivity test failed," and flashed the red light instead of the yellow one, with the alert tone beeping continually. I checked the reference manuals and followed the instructions, checking the lines and connections and clamps and pushing the buttons for a repeat check. Then I waited another 22 minutes or so for the machine to go through the next phase of the process to verify that the filter was fit to use, only to get the same warnings from the control panel. I can't recall for certain if it would allow for a third testing cycle or not, but either way the result was the same: "remove Pak" was the instruction on the digital read-out now. The box didn't pass muster.

"Remove Pak?" I exclaimed. "Then what?! We don't have another one!"

The cycler had a label with the toll-free number for NxStage customer service, and I called that. Some kind soul was at the other end of the telephone line in what was by now the middle of the night, ready and willing to answer my questions. He explained that sometimes this would happen, and to prevent any possible compromise to a patient's health, the computer in the control module was set to reject the filter if it didn't pass the series of tests set forth, and shut down the system until a new pak was installed. I advised him we had no other Paks and that our regular delivery wasn't scheduled until the following week.

"We'll ship a new Pak to you immediately tomorrow, by next-day UPS," he assured me. "In the meantime, you'll need to use the premixed bags for Larry's treatment."

OK. At least we had a Plan B on hand. The bags of premixed dialysate were one of the supply items that took up the most room on the closet shelves. They held 5 liters of fluid each, and were packed two bags to a box. The cardboard shipping boxes were reinforced on the sides with an additional layer of cardboard for protection. Even so, a few times the UPS driver would arrive with our monthly shipment and say, "This one doesn't look so good... " and display a box with a noticeably damp corner. He would also give us the opportunity to refuse that box, meaning it went back to the supplier.

Larry's treatments started out using 20 liters of dialysate, so a session with bags meant hanging four of them from the hooks of the IV-pole attached to the back of the machine. Five liters of fluid in a heavy-gauge plastic bag weigh about 11 pounds, and the pole was positioned about 6 feet high. The bags are flexible and have two small reinforced holes at the upper corners by which they hang from the hooks on the stainless steel bars at the top of the pole. At the bottom of each bag is a short plastic tube, protected by a screw-on plastic cap. Sometimes when I'd rip open the plastic sack in which a bag was encased before being put into the box for shipment, I'd find the plastic cap for this bag rolling around inside the sack. Because all connections were supposed to be made using sterile protocol (meaning: "don't touch the surfaces!"), I'd have to decide if this meant that the bag's contents—or at least the tube through which those contents would travel—had been compromised. Thinking back, this was probably something I should have asked the NxStage folks. Instead, I just got into the habit of checking the cap through the translucent sack before ripping it open, making sure it was tight enough not to fall off in the process.

Once the bags were hung up, I would remove each little cap and thread on a connecting tube from a set of six. The six tubes merged into two sets of three, and the two sets of three into one set that led to a warmer sack, which looks like a little clear vinyl pouch about 6 x 8 inches, comprising a number of horizontally zig-zagged chambers. The pouch (when flat) was placed into a warming device beside the cycler, and was used to bring the dialysate from the bags up to (or at least close to) body temperature, something the PureFlow cabinet is programmed to do for the big 60-liter saks of dialysate it holds. If you forget to turn the warmer on (as I did once), the patient's blood runs through the cartridge in the cycler and is surrounded by the room-temperature dialysate when it goes through the filter and is therefore returned to your patient in a much cooler state than when it left him. This is *not good*.

Many people who have dialysis in a treatment center will tell you it makes them cold. Larry got cold during treatment in center, and seemed to get even colder at home. I tend to keep the thermostat for the house set about 70 degrees year-round, so maybe the center was warmer than that. The connecting tubes from the catheter (or later his fistula) are only a few feet long, but in the course of those few feet they are exposed to room air; maybe this contributes to the cooling factor. But when the dialysate isn't heated sufficiently (or at all!) the chill can be rapid, and obviously, systemic. Larry felt like an ice cube, and I felt like a horrible person! Amidst chattering teeth and profuse apologies, I flipped the switch on the back of the heater to the "on" setting and piled on the blankets, grabbed a couple of heating pads to speed up the process from without, and warmed a towel in the microwave to apply to his chest and neck. The situation was remedied fairly quickly, but I never again forgot to check that the power supply was plugged in securely, and that the switch was in the "on" position if we were using bags for a treatment.

* * *

As I mentioned, NxStage sent a delivery each month by UPS. This included the PurePak filters, the Saks of dialysate concentrate (two Saks to a box), the premixed bags of dialysate, warmer sets, and the cartridges (six to a box) with the tubing and filter. We used one cartridge for each treatment, unless there was a malfunction, of which we experienced maybe two or three in the 3-1/2 years of dialysis. The Saks made 60 liters, so initially one Sak was sufficient quantity for three treatments, provided we completed those within the timeframe allowed: the control panel on the PureFlow cabinet was programmed to consider the dialysate in a Sak "expired" after 72 hours, and would shut down the flow from a Sak if that time limit was reached, even if this was in the middle of a treatment. It would also provide a warning on the digital screen at the start of a treatment if it was nearing that expiration time, so I could plan ahead and have a bag or two ready with the warming set and switch over to that if necessary to complete a session. It took more than 7 hours for the machine to make a Sak once I had one loaded in the cabinet, hooked up the lines, and pressed the buttons to commence the process. Afterward, there was a conductivity check, similar to the one for the Pak, and if the Sak failed this test three times, the control panel was likewise programmed to reject the use of it and required it to be drained. One drain cycle ran between 2 and 3 hours, and was insufficient to completely drain 60 liters of fluid, but it could lighten the bag enough for me to shut off the machine, clamp and disconnect the hoses, and lift the partially emptied plastic Sak from the stainless steel bin of the warming cabinet, carry it to the kitchen sink, cut it open and finish draining it.

As you've probably figured out, timing was sometimes a challenge. If you are a patient considering home hemodialysis and your care partner works a full-time job, put some consideration into this. Think about and discuss honestly and realistically how much of this process you'll be able to perform yourselves, and whether you have close friends or relatives who might be able to provide occasional help with the treatments or with other household duties. This is a stressful time, and a good support system may make a huge difference in your mental and emotional health.

*   *   *

As for those inventories, NxStage provided a helpful one-page chart on which I wrote the date and notations regarding the number of Saks, Paks, dialysate bags, warmer sets, and cartridges we had on hand. I typically faxed the sheet in to their customer service center, but I could also call them with the information. They'd calculate the order for shipment based on the doctor's orders for the number of treatments per week and the total number of liters of dialysate to be used each time. Because we lived so far away from our clinic location, they made sure we always had enough bags for at least a week's worth of treatments on hand, just in case. And if I failed to get the inventory sheet in by the appropriate date, we'd get an automated reminder call. If that didn't trigger some action by the next day or so, one of the customer service reps would call for the information. They were always very kind and did an excellent job of following through on whatever we needed from their company to keep up with Larry's treatments.

92

A typical monthly shipment from NxStage would include 3 or 4 boxes of cartridges, 4 or 5 boxes of "Saks" with dialysate concentrate, 2 large boxes with a PurePak each, the occasional box of warmer sets (with 24 to a box, that one lasted a while), and, depending on how many times during the month we'd used bags (if any) anywhere from 0 to 6 boxes of the premixed bags of dialysate solution. The UPS guy definitely got a workout when he delivered to our place. To anyone considering home hemodialysis: you might consider getting a dolly to move boxes. The UPS employee who made most of our deliveries at the time brought the boxes into the house and put them in whatever spot I requested, which was always some place on the ground floor. We had a substitute driver one time who wanted to just hand me all 17 boxes at the door, saying something about not being permitted to come inside. I didn't hesitate to let him know that wasn't going to fly.

Initially, some of the other supplies came through a medical supply company that delivered, but before long the routine changed to us picking up the peripheral supplies from the dialysis clinic at Larry's monthly visit. At some point in the week before that I'd make a chart on a tablet, listing all the items used other than those from NxStage: 10-mL plastic syringes with and without needles, 2x2 and 3x3 gauze pads, tape, bottles of heparin, latex gloves, face masks, alcohol wipes, saline bags, dialysis needle sets, etc. I'd check the calendar for the number of treatment days between the inventory date and the following month's clinic date. Next to each item I wrote down how many of that particular thing we used per treatment, then multiplied that times the number of treatments pending, and added that number to the next column labeled "# needed." In the middle column I inserted the inventory numbers to show "# on hand." Finally I subtracted column 2 from column 1 to get "# to order" in column 3. Then I typed up a list of the items in column 3 and either emailed or faxed it to Larry's nurse at the clinic, who would have his supplies together and ready to load when he arrived for his appointment. She would also include the test tube labels for the next month's lab tests, and more test tubes when needed.

Depending on the results of the most recent lab tests, Dr.

Winkelmeyer might prescribe a weekly shot of EPO, a very expensive medication that promotes the production of red blood cells and is often used to treat anemia in dialysis patients or those undergoing treatment for cancer. This we picked up from the clinic also, along with 1-mL syringes for administering the injections, and a cold pack if I'd forgotten to bring one along, because EPO has to be kept at a certain temperature to be effective.

Another item the clinic supplied was prescription-strength vitamin D capsules, when they were needed. Again, Dr. W. would make recommendations based on the monthly lab reports. We adhered to his advice religiously. If for some reason we felt a particular prescription or protocol was unnecessary or causing an adverse side effect, we would discuss it with him. He was always willing to listen to our concerns and explain his reasoning to both Larry and me.

* * *

The clinic in Columbia employs a social worker, and we found a true helper in Sarah Felmey. She sent some papers home with Larry soon after he began treatments there so I could fill them out and then return them to her. She then submitted these forms on Larry's behalf. The resulting benefit was that the premium for his Medicare supplement policy (at that time, $268 per month) was paid by the American Kidney Fund from that point forward. WOW!! This made a huge positive impact on our budget, which had been under considerable strain for many years, in a large part due to Larry's long-term health problems. Sarah also found a program that provided a one-time grant for assistance with our travel expenses back and forth for medical treatment and training. Over the course of the 3-1/2 years we worked with the clinic, she was a constant source of positive reassurance, empathy, and professional knowledge. Thank you, Sarah!

Another very nice lady at the clinic was Suzette Vos, the dietician. She sent monthly analysis reports of key numbers from the lab results, showing positives and negatives from the readings that reflected the quality of Larry's nutrition each month, with suggestions on how the negatives might be improved. She supplied samples of some specialty items that could help his protein levels when those were low, and coupons for the bottles of Ensure that she knew he preferred to eating breakfast. With her easy smile and gentle nature, Suzette encouraged but didn't nag, ever. What a sweetie!

Larry's prescriptions changed from time to time according to the variable lab results. When he first began dialysis he took Phoslo, a phosphorus binder, every time he ate something. After several months, however, he was able to discontinue this pill. Whether that was due to the efficiency of the treatments or his lack of appetite or a combination thereof, I don't know.

Very quickly after he started dialysis, the blood pressure medicine he'd taken for a long time was dropped from his list of medications, never to return.

When we began using the fistula in his arm, there was a prescription for Lidocaine and Prilocaine cream that Larry applied to the area 30 to 60 minutes before insertion of the needles. It usually helped to lessen the discomfort he felt during the process. Sometimes he would say he barely felt it when I oh-so-carefully threaded those 15-gauge needles into his vein, checked for flow, then taped everything into place. Other times I could tell by the controlled flinch and sharp intake of breath that it had hurt like hell. Geez, how I hated those times! I have always been a ninny about needles (just ask my mother!), sometimes becoming physically sick when, as a child, I thought I might have to get an injection, and even actually passing out when I had to have blood drawn as an adult.

More than once I told Larry: "There's something wrong with a treatment that requires a person to physically hurt their spouse in the process." Usually at this point there were tears streaming down my face, because I had just done that very thing. He would very gamely try to shrug it off and tell me not to worry about it, maybe even attempt to convince me that it really hadn't bothered him that much at all... but I knew this guy. I knew how much pain I'd seen him withstand in the past and how it had to be really bad before he'd ever show any outwardly visible sign that something hurt. The thought that I had been responsible for inflicting that level of pain on the love of my life was brutal, mentally and emotionally.

95

And for Larry, added to the physical pain was the mental/emotional challenge of trying to hide it and then reassure me that "it wasn't that bad." No fun.

On the flip side, there were definite advantages to performing his treatments at home.

He didn't need to drive 90 miles each way to the clinic three times a week. This became a truly good thing about 6 months later when his back "gave way," because there were a lot of days after that when he physically could not have made the drive, and I certainly couldn't take off work three days a week to drive him there, wait through the treatment, then drive him home, even if his back could have tolerated the journey.

Instead of the vinyl upholstered recliner in the center, he sat on his own reclining sofa or La-Z-Boy rocker/recliner, in the comfort of his own living room, where he could sleep or read a magazine or watch TV or visit with me or a friend who might drop by. The reclined position is mandatory, in case of a drop in blood pressure, so that you can raise the patient's feet and lower their head to assist in stabilizing them. Nurse Lisa had told us this beforehand; we had the sofa already, and got the chair later. Larry much preferred being at home to the option of being in the treatment center.

Health-wise, the in-home treatments meant Larry wasn't exposed to as many germs as he might have been in-center. Although the dialysis technicians and nurses take every precaution to keep things sterile at the clinic, it's impossible to control who might be coming in there with a virus or infection of which they might not even be aware, and colds and flu can spread quickly. At home we had a little more control over who came in, and politely discouraged visits from anyone who was less than healthy. These extra steps of protection were important to us.

Having dialysis five or six times a week also helped keep Larry's fluid levels under better control, so that his blood pressure didn't get too high between treatments, and the fluctuations in his weight due to excess fluid were less severe. These, in turn, equaled less strain on his heart. This is important for all patients, obviously, and because Larry had already suffered one heart attack and undergone quintuple bypass surgery several years prior to starting

96

dialysis, we were highly sensitive to this advantage.

At the time of this writing, an Internet search for "home hemodialysis" located three companies that offer these programs. NxStage is the one we worked with (through a DaVita dialysis clinic). According to my search information, the other two companies require a reverse-osmosis water supply for their machines. I'll admit to being familiar with the concept, but ignorant of the details. Another generalized article I read about the process of in-home hemodialysis indicated that of the patients currently on dialysis, only 0.4% are using home hemodialysis (commonly called HHD). Nurse Lisa at DaVita explained to me that as the baby boomer population ages, the number of people requiring dialysis is expected to rise rapidly. Dialysis clinics could become more crowded than ever. The goal of better patient care (meaning improved quality of life combined with fewer adverse effects at a decreased overall cost), appears to be pointing toward HHD where appropriate. In spite of the challenges we faced, I am convinced it was the right treatment for Larry, and HHD is a wonderful alternative to in-center dialysis. Just be prepared to commit a lot of time to the process, be meticulous with your organization, and don't skip treatments!

13
TESTING, TESTING...

Although dialysis removes enough toxins from a person's bloodstream to keep him or her alive, it doesn't necessarily allow the person to feel what you might term "good." I'd read what I could find about kidney transplants, and Larry and I agreed to pursue this idea as a possible long-term treatment option for him.

On Wednesday, May 28, 2008, I called the Transplant Institute at a major hospital in Kansas City. It was more than 100 miles from our home, and we prefer to drive in smaller towns, but I was willing to explore this option if it would best help my husband. I spoke with "Nicki" who told me we'd have to enroll in pre-transplant education classes, and that a program coordinator would call me for Larry's insurance information and, if it proved acceptable, they'd sign us up for the class and send some booklets for us to read.

A full week later on June 5, I called there again, since "Carmen" had never returned my call. I was transferred to her extension, and she took the information on Larry's policies from Medicare and his supplement. She told me she'd fax an authorization form that would enable them to obtain information from the DaVita clinic, and that a doctor there would review the chart when they'd compiled more details. I asked some specific questions about their success rates, the ratio of transplants performed from living donors vs. deceased donors, and the potential for a combined kidney-pancreas transplant for Larry. Carmen was not encouraging. She said Larry might be considered for that program, but his age was a negative factor (he was 58 years and 8 months to the day). They preferred to keep these dual-transplant patients under 60, and by the time he went through all the required testing, and then waited for a donor, she predicted he'd be over the limit of their guidelines.

So, I called University Hospital in Columbia, Missouri, and left a message for Alice Misfeldt, RN, the transplant nurse coordinator, asking her to call me regarding their program. Within 27 hours, she did so. I asked about kidney-pancreas transplants, but was told that at that time they were doing only kidney transplants, not the two organs together. I also inquired about islet cell transplants, in which islet cells from a healthy person's pancreas are transplanted into a diabetic patient to sort of "jump-start" the patient's ability to process sugar. (That's an enormous over-simplification, I'm sure!) No, they weren't doing those procedures either. She recommended we talk more in depth with Dr. Winkelmeyer and find out what he thought might be the best path for Larry to pursue.

My next call, then, was to Dr. W's office. He wasn't in, but nurse practitioner Anita Cox was, and I was happy to talk with her. Anita had known us for a long time and was highly familiar with Larry's history. My impression from her was that although the kidney-pancreas surgeries and their implied "cure" for diabetes sounded promising, they were still considered more risky than the kidney transplant alone. She urged us to "try for the kidney now," and assured us that Dr. Winkelmeyer would send a letter of referral to the transplant team at University Hospital.

In mid-June 2008, Larry received a letter from Nurse Alice, along with some brochures to read. The letter indicated she would call us soon and set up the initial appointments to screen Larry for eligibility in the transplant program.

Our first drive to University Hospital that year was on Tuesday, July 8. A letter had been sent out on June 27, confirming the date and times for this preliminary evaluation. I had printed a list of potential questions to ask from a website I'd recently read, and had also perused the Medicare benefits handbook to familiarize myself with what costs were covered under that plan.

A social worker met with us first. She confirmed that Medicare would pick up the tab for a kidney transplant, including doctors and hospital fees, lab tests, and three types of immunosuppressant drugs. Other medications would be covered under the Part D prescription plan we'd chosen. She suggested that for the coming years, we investigate the options of those Part D plans that had coverage within the "Donut Hole" coverage gap, during which most plans cover no drug costs. Some of the required meds were available in generic form, but depending on the individual patient's needs and reactions, these were not always feasible, and the annual cost of the necessary prescriptions could add up quickly.

The social worker also explained that a kidney donation from a live donor often provided better results, and that if needed, she'd help us research possible grants to assist with lost wages for such a donor if and when that time came.

Step 2 that day was a meeting with Alice Misfeldt, the pre-kidney transplant nurse coordinator we'd talked with by phone, and a transplant surgeon. They indicated Larry's cardio function would be the first thing to be tested, and that his heart doctor from previous years could do the honors in that regard. After that, there would be blood work, x-rays, and other tests to verify his general health. The surgeon mentioned the six markers of compatibility that were checked for matching whenever a donor organ became available. Larry's A+ blood type meant he could receive a kidney from a donor with either type A or type O blood; the typical wait time in our area was 18 months to 2 years. After transplant surgery, the doctor told us, most of his patients spend 2 to 3 days in ICU, and 7 to 14 days in the hospital before going home, then are closely monitored for signs of rejection of the organ. He checked the abdominal scars Larry had from his previous surgery (after the car accident, when they had to repair his spleen and liver) and reassured us that those should not pose a problem. He also warned us that the immune suppression drugs can increase one's susceptibility to cancer. But overall, he was upbeat, positive, and encouraging.

The third visit was with a nephrologist, Dr. K. He told us about a new insulin pump that would come with a glucose sensor and could be preset with a range for alarms to indicate high and low blood sugar readings. He listened to Larry's heart and lungs and confirmed that Dr. Spaedy's approval would be needed before they could go any further in the process. If the patient's heart isn't strong enough to endure the surgery, the team would obviously be remiss to proceed!

* * *

Dr. Spaedy's office is in the Missouri Heart Center, across from Boone Hospital in Columbia, Missouri. The team there does a good job juggling a lot of patients while maintaining a great reputation for quality care. I called there immediately after our interviews with the transplant team, and explained what was going on.

"When was your husband's last visit with Dr. Spaedy?" the scheduling secretary asked.

"Well, that was probably in the Spring of 2000", I told her. "I don't have the exact date handy."

"2000?" she sounded perplexed. "He hasn't seen the doctor in over 8 years?"

"Uh, no. Larry had bypass surgery in February of 2000, and was cleared by the surgeon several weeks later, and I think he saw Dr. Spaedy then, too. Doc told us to call him if we needed him, and... well, we haven't needed him! Larry's heart has been doing just fine. He just needs Dr. Spaedy to vouch for that to the transplant team before they'll put him on the list for a kidney."

There was a long pause on the other end of the line. I got the feeling she thought maybe Larry hadn't seen *any* doctors in 8 years, which was far from true!

"He's been seeing his nephrologist, Dr. Winkelmeyer, regularly all this time, and Dr. Winkelmeyer is the one who referred him to Dr. Spaedy when his heart was acting up," I offered.

"OK, well, the doctor is going to need to see Larry again before he'll offer any opinions like that."

"Yes, I understand. May we schedule that please?" (I think this girl was new!)

She checked with the doctor or his nurse and came back on the line to report that Larry would need to have a cardiac stress test, and they could see him on July 17 for that.

The cardiac stress test can be done on a treadmill, or through a chemically-induced process that mimics the effects of strenuous physical activity. Larry had had the treadmill-type test back in 1998 after his heart attack. I was in the room, and heard the beeps of the monitor getting closer together as the machine went faster and the incline steeper, and then the alarm chiming as it sent him into another little "episode." The technician hit the stop button as Dr. Spaedy sprayed liquid nitro under Larry's tongue and they each took hold of one of his arms to ease him back down into the waiting wheelchair parked behind him. This was a little scary, to say the least. He'd repeated the same type of test before his bypass surgery, when he was feeling draggy and sluggish again. But between then and now, arthritis had taken a toll on his joints and Larry questioned whether his back would tolerate the treadmill test.

"Better make it the chemical kind this time," he said.

So they did, but he didn't like it. "That hurt," Larry said afterward.

The stress test showed a slight abnormality, which prompted an angiogram on July 28 at the same location. This gave Dr. Spaedy a peek at the arteries and the heart and just how things were working inside Larry's chest.

"Of the five bypasses that were done in 2000, four of them are great and doing exactly what they're supposed to. The fifth one apparently branched over to a smaller vein and that's why we got the abnormal reading on the stress test," Dr. Spaedy told us afterward. "It's OK, though; the other four are sufficient, Larry's heart muscle is strong, and I see no reason to intervene at this point."

He also told us he didn't think this condition should preclude the possibility of a kidney transplant, and that he would fax his findings to the transplant team and to Dr. Winkelmeyer.

OK! Round One down!

* * *

The results must have reached the team fairly quickly after that, because we soon received a letter dated July 31, 2008, advising us of more tests scheduled for Larry on Friday, August 8. He was to report to University Hospital at 7:40 am, which made for an early drive to Columbia that day. With the gas tank in the old Suburban topped off beforehand, we tried to allow 2 hours for the trip, especially when we had to find a spot in their parking garage and then make our way to a certain spot inside the hospital.

Nurse Alice met us in the lobby and brought a packet with the day's requisitions and a map of their facility, marking the locations of the appointments to assist us. First they performed an Abdominal/Renal Carotid and Lower Extremity ultrasound in radiology. Then a laboratory technician drew blood, filling 14 test tubes for various workups.

"Did you leave me any?" Larry asked the lady.

"A little!" she said. The last item that day was a chest x-ray, and we were out of there before noon. If this was Round Two... well, gee, that wasn't so bad.

The next letter, for Round 3, was faxed to us on August 18 and disclosed Larry's next appointments for Thursday, August 21. (I have a fax machine at home because of my work.) He was to have an MRI exam of his abdomen at 10:15 am in the imaging center across town from the hospital, followed by a 4 pm visit with Dr. T. at the clinic near the center. This doctor's focus was on gastrointestinal issues, and getting clearance from him was the next step necessary to move any further along in the transplant approval process. The notes I kept don't include this day's appointments; it's possible that Larry went by himself. The paperwork in the file indicates he had a CT scan of the abdominal area instead of an MRI. So, Round 3 didn't seem so bad.

My steno pad does include notes from a meeting in the dialysis clinic on Monday, August 25, and indicate that the Epogen he was receiving was helping his hemoglobin levels, albeit slowly, and that the nurse performed a tuberculin skin test. Another item written down that day was: "Do not lift more than 10 pounds w/ left arm – ever" because of the fistula. We had also been warned never to allow anyone to use that arm for blood pressure readings. This proved to be something I had to be really vigilant about during Larry's subsequent hospital stays. Having it in the record, posted on the wall behind his left shoulder, on a wristband... none of those methods was 100% foolproof. Nurses and their aides are usually kept very busy, and it's easy to become distracted when someone else pops their head into the room with a question just as they're about to take someone's vital signs. This is one reason I believe it's important for patients to have an advocate, especially if they are on pain medication or otherwise sedated for any reason.

Also on August 25 a surgeon who specializes in veins and arteries and their processes, performed a fistulagram on Larry. This is a procedure similar to an angiogram, in which a small tube with a camera is threaded through the artery to examine the status of the fistula from inside. He then did a small outpatient revision to the vein on September 10, and told us the fistula should be ready for use a week later.

The next day at 10 AM, Dr. T. called regarding the findings of the MRI. He said it showed a lesion or mass on Larry's liver, and that the most common cause of something like this was metastatic cancer, meaning cancer that had originated elsewhere and migrated to this spot. He ordered a colonoscopy to begin investigating the issue, because it is a lower-risk procedure than a biopsy. The mass could be benign, he said, but he didn't know yet. Besides, a colonoscopy would be part of the normal transplant screening process anyway. Oh, and they'd draw more blood the same day, for more tests.

Obviously that was a scary conversation. Who doesn't hear the "C" word and get scared? Well, my husband appeared to be one of those people. He was so nonchalant. "It's not cancer," he told me in such a calm tone, the same as if he was telling me "it's not raining today."

"You think?" I queried.

"Yeah, I think," he responded. "I think I would feel it if it were cancer. Don't worry."

"But I do worry," I told him. "It's my job to worry."

He slowly shook his head in the negative. "Don't worry," he repeated. "You know what I always tell you: 'don't worry until it's time to worry', right?"

"But what if it *is* time?!"

Cool as a cucumber, he just smiled and shook his head again.

"It's not. Believe me."

* * *

So on September 16, in addition to the monthly clinic visit at DaVita at 8:30 am, we returned to University Hospital for another blood draw. This time I asked what they were testing for exactly, and was told a "CMP" (complete metabolic panel) and a CA 19-9 (more about that in a moment). At 10:30 Larry checked in for the colonoscopy. They found and removed a polyp, and the lab report 2 days later pronounced it benign. The doctor who conducted the test recommended it be repeated in 5 years.

Round 4 was over.

When we got home I looked up the CA 19-9 blood test on the Internet and got at least a little scared all over again. Carbohydrate antigen 19-9 (also called cancer antigen 19-9) is a tumor marker that may be elevated in some types of gastrointestinal (GI) cancers, such as those of the colon, esophagus, pancreas, and liver. A higher-than-normal number on this test can also result from cirrhosis of the liver, pancreatitis, and either diseased or blocked bile ducts. At least one article I read indicated the test often gives false impressions, as in high numbers when there is no cancer, or even low numbers when cancer is present.

"OK, God," I prayed, "whatever it is You have in store for us, we know You'll be with us throughout. It's hard for us humans to admit we're not in control. The truth is, we aren't, and deep down I know that. I can try to control my reactions, though, and ask Your help in that. Please help me not to react with fear, but with confidence and faith, and with the loving support Larry needs, no matter what. Amen."

* * *

The follow-up appointment to this was on October 8, 2008, with a nurse practitioner. She explained to us that the CT scan had been reviewed with a radiologist, and that it revealed two spots on Larry's liver. One of these was about 2 centimeters square and was puckering the liver's surface. The CA 19-9 blood test done on August 21 showed a reading of 200; the repeat test conducted on October 16 said 253. A "normal" test result would be 0 to 37. She confirmed that this tumor marker is specific to the GI tract. To investigate the areas of concern, they had scheduled a biopsy procedure called "fine needle aspiration: or FNA. She explained that Larry would be sedated and given a local anesthetic for the process. Afterward he would need to lie on his side for 3 to 4 hours before we could go home. Laboratory results would be expected 5 to 7 days after that. The nurse also said an endoscopic ultrasound likely would be scheduled for some time after the biopsy but might not be necessary, depending on the findings. And once again, they drew blood.

So this was Round 5.

On October 22, with Larry in the "twilight zone," so to speak, an interventional radiologist used ultrasound guidance and a very long, hollow needle to obtain cell samples of the 2-cm lesion on Larry's liver. He told me afterward the spot was just under the liver capsule, and while it didn't look too menacing to him from the view available, the laboratory results would tell us more.

My printed copy of the lab report saying "benign" is dated October 28. Funny how a six-letter word like that can open our airways for a deeper breath, isn't it?

*   *   *

Meanwhile, on October 23, another fistulagram showed a narrowing in a portion of the vein, which was opened with a balloon procedure at the same time. This proved to be the last time the fistula would need outside intervention, and we used it exclusively and successfully for Larry's dialysis treatments for the next 3 years.

The next bump in the road involved Larry's back. He had seen a local doctor over the summer for a flare-up of back pain, and even tried a few chiropractic visits, but with little success. He had been diagnosed with degenerative disk disease in the spring of 2005, when a doctor told him he had 3 collapsed disks at the mid to lower level of his spine, and was living with a lot of pain from the residual effects of all those broken bones over the years. By 2008 Darvocet had become one of his regular prescriptions to help with the pain — "help" being the key word. The pain was always there, at least in the background. Larry had not been pain free for many years.

About 3 am on Friday, October 31, 2008, while simply turning over in bed, something in his back gave way, and Larry woke with a loud cry of distress. The pain was severe and relentless. There was a bottle of pain pills next to the bed, and I fetched one of the muscle-relaxing tablets that had been prescribed for him earlier. He made it through most of the day, but finally by late afternoon agreed to an ER visit. We arrived in the emergency room in Sedalia by 5 pm. In addition to the back pain, he mentioned knifing pains in his belly that radiated around to the left.

The ER staff put in an IV and infused pain and nausea meds. They drew blood and took an x-ray, which was inconclusive. His white blood cell count was elevated at 13,800 (normal range being around 4,300 to 10,800). The doctor suspected a kidney infection and prescribed an antibiotic for that, and Vicodin instead of Darvocet for the pain. We were to call Dr. Winkelmeyer on Monday for follow-up.

By Monday not much was improved. The abdominal pains were radiating to the back on both sides, and Anita, the nurse practitioner who worked with Dr. W., ordered a CT scan. Like the x-ray at the emergency room, this test didn't reveal any great mysteries. Anita did say "no more Vicodin," because the stronger narcotic could cause constipation, and changed the antibiotic to one more friendly to Larry's kidneys.

The following Saturday, November 8, we went to the ER at Boone Hospital in Columbia. Larry's severe pain had been continuous from the early hours of October 31, and he'd been on antibiotics for 8 days with no sign of improvement. Any activity was causing shortness of breath, and we needed to figure out why and what to do about it. They did more blood work, more x-rays, another urine test, another CT scan. The white cell count was still around 13,000, but we were told this was "not an infectious cell and could be from his high blood glucose reading of 557." Larry delivered the appropriate amount of insulin from his pump to counteract this.

After 3 to 4 hours in the little windowless room, we were told that this all was a result of the degenerative disk and joint disease. At least one spot in Larry's back was bone-on-bone, with no joint cushioning left. They'd also found a small incisional hernia in his belly, but didn't feel it was related to the excruciating pain he was experiencing. The ER doctor recommended some epidural injections, which would be scheduled through the radiology department, and wrote a prescription for Percocet (stronger than either the Darvocet or the Vicodin) for pain control, and another for something to counteract the Percocet's digestive effects.

The first epidural injection took place the following Tuesday, November 11, at Boone Hospital. Steroidal medications were infused in the L3-L4 area of Larry's spine. Afterward he told me it "hurt like hell."

But as they say, The Show Must Go On. Larry still wanted a kidney transplant and had to complete the screening to get on the waiting list. So that same day we stopped by University Hospital for the "pre-op" chest x-ray, EKG, and (of course) blood work required for Round 6, which began the next day at 7 am. The endoscopic ultrasound took place first. This involved another trip to the "twilight zone," and then a little flexible tube with an ultrasound attachment was sent down Larry's throat and through his stomach all the way to the small intestine to check out his liver, pancreas, spleen, etc. We were given printed reports with both color and black-and-white pictures and text describing a dilated side branch of the pancreatic duct and a "prominent" ampulla, which is the joining of the bile duct and the main pancreatic duct. Tissue samples of the ampulla were taken for laboratory analysis.

In the afternoon, with Larry mostly awake, we drove across Columbia to an imaging center for MRI and MRCP (magnetic resonance cholangeopancreatography) scans of the same area. Being flat on his back in the machine long enough for this test was no picnic, but he soldiered through. The technicians gave us a CD with images to give to the doctor, and told us the nurse would be calling with the next appointment date.

As you might imagine, this was all a little nerve-racking. Every little step we took seemed to lead to more steps down these side paths, and it was difficult to tell whether any progress was being made toward the goal of getting a kidney for Larry. He'd been on dialysis for more than 7 months now, and still didn't even seem close to being approved to get on the list. And the types of things they had to rule out (understandably!) were getting a little scary.

Late in the day on Friday, November 14, a nurse called to report that the biopsy samples taken during the endoscopic ultrasound were benign. The doctor would be reviewing the report the following week and would call with his recommendations. She also told me the CA 19-9 blood test numbers can show elevations from all tumors, not just those that are malignant. Nurse Angie called again on Monday afternoon to confirm that the MRI had shown nothing to indicate cancer in Larry's digestive system. Still, he was to follow-up with the doctor in clinic on December 11.

Why? I don't know.

Why the wait? I don't know.

Did I ask those questions of Angie? Looking back... yes, probably.

Did she know? Probably not. Bless her, she was just relaying news that she knew we'd want to hear. And Round 6 was complete.

* * *

We found out that Larry had to be back in Columbia on December 4 to have his fistula checked one more time (just to be sure) and then to have the Permacath taken out. I called the digestive health clinic, and they were able to move the appointment from the 11th to the 4th, to save us a trip. The Permacath removal was a bit painful, Larry said, but not too bad. A sterile bandage was placed over the holes where the tubes had exited his chest since April, but no stitches were required.

At the clinic with Dr. P., we were provided a copy of the MRI report. It mentioned the duct issues the doctor had discussed with us, and recommended an endoscopic ultrasound (!). It also called Larry's kidneys "atrophic" — no surprise there, given that he'd been on dialysis for months. The abnormality along the edge of his liver was remarked on, along with the small hernia. The only news we hadn't heard before was the presence of stones in his gallbladder. The doctor would discuss that with the transplant team and find out if this was an issue, and let us know.

But before we left they drew blood for yet another CA 19-9 test.

The following Tuesday, December 9, a nurse called from the GI doctors' office. The CA 19-9 test now showed a reading of 123, which was lower than before but still higher than normal. Dr. T. and Dr. P. had agreed to refer Larry to a general surgeon to see if his gallbladder should be removed. The nurse scheduled the

109

appointment while I was on the phone with her: December 22, with Dr. Nicole Fearing, at the University Hospital Clinics. We figured that would constitute Round 7.

* * *

Meanwhile, Larry's back pain that had turned so severe on Halloween day was not abating. The epidural injection at Boone Hospital's radiology department hadn't made any difference, and he ended up back in Columbia on December 11 anyway, for an MRI of his lumbar spine at Boone Hospital. We'd been referred to a pair of neurosurgeons across the street from the hospital, in the building between Dr. Winkelmeyer's office and the DaVita clinic, right next door to Dr. Spaedy's. Nurse Lisa Baker told me these two were the best in town. When I called to make an appointment for Larry the office manager explained that either doctor would want the MRI for reference before a first appointment, and she was very helpful in getting it set up right away.

But by December 22 when I drove Larry to his monthly DaVita clinic visit, he felt horrible. The pain was interrupting his sleep and had annihilated his appetite. For someone who didn't have any extra weight to lose, this was concerning. Nurse Lisa could see it etched across his face and called Dr. Winkelmeyer right away. She then packed us off to the ER across the street at Boone, assuring us she'd call Dr. Fearing's office at University Hospital to let them know why we weren't going to make that visit.

In the emergency room Larry told them of the excruciating pain in his back and stomach, and that the Percocet was not helping. We hadn't heard back from the neurosurgeon's office regarding the MRI scan that had been done 11 days earlier. I tried to clarify to the doctor on duty that we weren't just there for more drugs or better drugs or different drugs to mask the pain... we wanted answers. We wanted something to be fixed! The ER doctor found the MRI images in their computer system and consulted with Dr. Winkelmeyer by phone. The images did not justify surgery on Larry's back if other methods would help, and a pain management specialist was called in. What followed was one of the most

110

frustrating experiences we'd ever had in that hospital.

Dr. X was not brand new, but younger than us by quite a bit. He seemed confident, maybe in the extreme. Not unfriendly, but glib and a bit crude. He proposed an epidural injection. We reminded him Larry had received one of those on November 11 and it had not alleviated the pain.

"Yes, but I didn't do that injection," was his reply; as if no one but himself was capable of doing it correctly. He also made a rather snide remark questioning why we would allow anyone from the radiology department to perform such an important task? Well, gee, we just did what was recommended, and the ER doctor we'd seen that time had recommended it! Dr. X went on to talk about various methods of treating back pain, including the deadening of nerves in the area, but cautioned that if the wrong nerve was put out of commission by mistake, "then you're just hosed."

Those were his exact words.

I was appalled. Not because I don't use blue language on occasion, but because I expected a certain level of professionalism from the medical professionals with whom we dealt, and because this guy had just met us a few minutes beforehand. He was really taking some liberties, in my opinion.

However, Larry was in no condition to be waiting for yet another opinion, and I was desperate to obtain help for him in whatever form it took, so we agreed to try Dr. X's plan. He prescribed a 50-mcg fentanyl pain patch, explaining that it was designed to release the medicine transdermally over a period of 3 days, and wrote a prescription for a month's supply of these. Fentanyl is another opium derivative, stronger than the Percocet tablets.

The next morning we met Dr. X in the pain clinic on the other side of the hospital. The epidural injection he performed hurt Larry worse than the one the month before. This one was in the L2-L3 area. After realizing that even with the local anesthetic he'd not been able to better the issue, Dr. X agreed to refer Larry to Dr. Ryan (one of the two neurosurgeons across the street we'd been trying to see) for another opinion. He would also order a bone scan and wanted to see Larry again in 3 to 4 weeks.

I didn't tell him not to hold his breath on that one. But I thought about it.

* * *

The season was so hectic and our living space so disorganized and crowded with dialysis supplies that no Christmas tree went up that year. As it turned out, it would be 2011 before a Christmas tree would return to the living room of our home. I didn't try to send out cards, and barely got presents wrapped because there were too few hours in my weeks. But just the same, Christmas came, as did New Year's. We stayed on schedule with Larry's treatments and didn't try to fit in any trips to see family. We just couldn't, time-wise, and Larry didn't feel up to any more travel than it took to get him back and forth to Columbia for the medical appointments.

A letter arrived dated December 31, confirming Larry's first appointment with Dr. Terry Ryan for January 21, 2009. Dr. Ryan talked with us and did some basic tests to measure Larry's strength and range of motion. He'd looked at the lower back images but told us he wanted another MRI, this time of the cervical spine, or neck area. He would also confer with Dr. Winkelmeyer before making any definitive plans for treatment, to be sure things stayed within bounds of the diabetes and dialysis issues.

We went out to the office manager's area. Dr. Ryan told Sue, the manager, what the next step needed to be, and she prepared to call Boone's radiology department to schedule the MRI.

"Do you think there's any chance whatsoever they might be able to fit that in today?" I asked. "It's a 90-mile drive each way.."

"Oh my, well, let's just see what we can do about that!" Sue had such a friendly, upbeat manner, it made calls and visits to that office an enjoyable experience.

And whether it was string-pulling, Sue's good working relationship with the scheduler across the street, or Divine Intervention, somehow Larry got the MRI done that day.

We returned to see Dr. Ryan again on January 30, where he showed us the images on a good-sized screen. There were bulging discs in Larry's neck at the C3-C4, C4-C5, and C5-C6 levels, putting pressure on his spinal cord. He recommended surgery to

112

remove the disks and stabilize the vertebrae with a plate and bone graft material taken from Larry's hip. The procedure is abbreviated as an ACDF, short for Anterior Cervical Discectomy and Fusion. He estimated 3 hours in the operating room and 1 to 2 days in the hospital, and told Larry he'd need to wear a cushioned support collar for a month afterward. After that he might be referred to physical therapy. But first (you guessed it) there was more blood work, a chest x-ray, and an EKG before Larry could be admitted to the hospital to have this done. The surgery was scheduled for Thursday, February 5.

* * *

Lest we forget Round 7 in the transplant screening process, the visit with Dr. Fearing had been reset for Monday, February 2. She examined Larry's belly and referred to the MRI and EUS (endoscopic ultrasound) reports confirming multiple stones in his gallbladder, and told us the organ should be removed, and why. A gallbladder with stones is more likely to flare up with inflammation or infection than one without. If it might have to be taken out anyway, it was safer to do so before Larry received a kidney (and the accompanying immune-suppressing drugs) than after. An infected gallbladder could be dangerous for someone on the necessary medications to prevent organ rejection. His slight build made a laparoscopic procedure probable, as opposed to a longer incision and a more painful recovery. Dr. Fearing told us to get the neck/back problems addressed first, heal up from that, and then call her to schedule the next surgery.

* * *

Early in the day on February 5 we arrived at Boone Hospital for the ACDF. The "anterior" part meant access was gained through the front of Larry's neck (to the right of center), rather than the back. I had trimmed his usually-full beard to an acceptable level so that it didn't have to be shaved. The incision proved to be surprisingly short—maybe 3 inches. Strips of surgical tape held it closed. Dr. Ryan assured me the surgery went just as he'd planned. After recovery, Larry was taken to a regular hospital room where he slept most of the rest of that day.

113

The next morning a physical therapist came in with the Miami "J" collar for neck support. It snugged into place with Velcro strips. Larry was advised to wear this whenever he was up walking around, while traveling, and while sleeping for the next 4 weeks until he saw Dr. Ryan for follow-up. The therapist walked around with Larry and made sure he could safely navigate the halls and some stairs. Then the hospital sent us home.

X-rays taken March 4 and again on April 29 showed the bones were mending well. The incision had healed very quickly and left such a thin scar that it was almost undetectable unless you knew what to look for and where, especially when Larry's beard grew back to normal length. Dr. Ryan wrote an order for physical therapy, and Larry met the therapist in Windsor three times a week. Sometimes, though, Larry wasn't able to make all of his appointments. In addition to the fentanyl patch, he often needed Percocet for the "break-through" pain in his back. As narcotics, these were prescribed and authorized by his doctor, and Larry was careful not to take more of them than he needed. In fact, he tried to stretch the doses out as far apart as he could tolerate. The pain medicines were playing havoc with his digestion and some days he just wasn't up to leaving the house.

* * *

Two months after the ACDF Larry felt that he was ready to tackle the gallbladder issue. He saw Dr. Fearing for pre-op on May 11 and went through the standard EKG, chest x-ray, and blood draw. Surgery was scheduled for May 26.

The day arrived and we checked in early in the morning. Dr. Fearing met with us in the pre-op area and asked if we had any last-minute questions.

"Do you pray before you cut?" I quizzed.

"You know, I pray every morning on my way to work that all my surgeries will go well, but if you'd like to pray right now about this one, I'll be happy to join hands and pray with you."

And so we did. We liked this lady already, but after that we were really impressed with the way she personally cared for her patients.

The laparoscopic procedure went just fine. Larry spent one night in the hospital and was released the next day.

With a follow-up visit to Dr. Fearing on June 15, Round 7 was finally complete.

14
ON THE LIST

A letter dated June 19, 2009, from Alice Misfeldt, Transplant Nurse Coordinator, began:

"Congratulations! You are now listed on our kidney transplant waiting list."

The letter went on to confirm the telephone numbers they had on file to reach us, explained the blood sample they'd need each month for cross-matching, and gave a brief description of what would happen when a match became available.

How to describe our emotions at that point?! We were thrilled with the prospect of life without dialysis. But we were also sobered and sad at the thought that this wonderful possibility for us would come at the expense of someone else, that a donor organ for Larry would mean some family, somewhere, had just lost someone very special. We did not take this lightly.

* * *

Although Larry's name was added to The List in June, he wasn't "active" on it until 6 weeks after the gallbladder removal surgery. Nurse Alice explained that if an organ matches more than one potential recipient in the area, the first call goes to the patient with the most accumulated days of waiting. "Inactive-status" patients still build days in this count, they're just not eligible to receive an organ while they are inactive. Another letter was sent confirming that Larry's "active" status began July 7, 2009. It was one day short of a year from that first set of appointments at University Hospital to begin the screening.

* * *

Ironically, reaching the 1-year mark in the process of getting onto the list meant it was time to start over with some of those tests. Dr. Spaedy was asked to verify cardiac clearance again. An office visit on July 29 was followed on the 30th with an echocardiogram. A painless procedure, a technician uses an ultrasound machine to check the electrical and muscular functions of the heart muscle and blood flow. The follow-up letter Dr. Spaedy sent (with a copy to the transplant team) called the results "excellent." He also wrote that Larry's heart muscle was very strong and that the valves were all working normally. Great news!

Those same 2 days Larry also saw Dr. Ryan again about the continuous back pain that had magnified exponentially the previous autumn. The neck surgery in January had helped somewhat. Dr. Ryan noted that Larry's grip was improved and he was able to sit up and stand straighter than before. But an MRI done on the first of July showed more narrowing in the disc spaces at L1-L2 and L3-L4. A bone scan at Boone Hospital was ordered for the next day. It showed a "hot spot" in the costovertebral joint where Larry's lowest ribs joined his spine. On August 7 Dr. Ryan put steroid injections in both sides of this area. There was so much relief from the local anesthetic that we went out to dinner afterward, and Larry actually ate! Unfortunately, the relief was brief—only a few weeks.

*　*　*

September 8, 2009, marked the removal of a cataract from Larry's left eye. In spite of the other numerous health problems, this brief surgery went very well. The fact that his vision was still very good after 55 years of diabetes was nothing short of a miracle.

"Did it hurt?" I asked after the procedure was done.

"No, not really," Larry told me. "A little uncomfortable, but not sharp pain."

When we arrived back home he noticed a bath towel hanging on a rack in the bathroom. He patted the terry cloth fabric lightly, as if it might be fragile.

"Wow, that's really white!" he marveled. His voice sounded pleasantly surprised, but I couldn't really understand why.

"Um, yeah, it is," I agreed, puzzled. "What color was it this morning?"

"Yellow."

"Yellow?"

"Yeah, yellow!"

"Wow."

He nodded. "Amazing!" was all he could say.

I nodded, my eyebrows still halfway up my forehead. "Amazing," I agreed.

Now and then, our days held a *nice* surprise. This was one of those days.

* * *

Jennifer and BJ had the same hectic schedules as most young working couples with four small children at home. With BJ working days driving a concrete truck and Jennifer putting in nights at the Schreiber plant in Clinton, Missouri, the few hours they had together over the weekends were all they had to squeeze in family visits and outings. They were very careful not to come over when any of them were sick, to avoid subjecting Larry to germs. Not only did they want to scrupulously avoid passing him a cold or flu virus, they also didn't want to get in the way of him being ready for a kidney if one became available.

But one Saturday that fall, when everyone was healthy and even Larry was feeling pretty good, the family came by to visit. As the afternoon faded into early evening, I began to get things ready for the dialysis treatment. Megan was about 3½ years old and was highly interested in the procedure. Her daddy advised her to stay back out of the way, but I could see her straining her neck to look over the edge of the cushions at what was happening around Papa's end of the couch. With his permission, I asked her if she'd like to help. Her deep brown eyes were shining with excitement as she nodded an emphatic yes.

"OK, then, first go wash your hands really well with soap and warm water."

She did, and came running back in.

"I'm ready!"

"Good job! Now here's some stuff that helps make your hands even cleaner," I told her, and showed her the pump dispenser of antibacterial gel. She knew how to operate that and followed my directions to rub it around all over her hands and between her fingers, just as we'd been taught at the clinic.

Megan seemed thrilled to take the chart to Papa with the flowsheet for recording the treatment details, and to get him the digital thermometer and push the button to turn it on. He let her push buttons on the blood pressure meter, too, and asked her to find the lidocaine cream tube in the little box of supplies on the end table nearby. As I opened the drawers of the plastic supply cabinet, I'd tell her how many of each item to take out and where to place it in our work area. Having a purpose in the process was making her very happy, so I kept thinking a step ahead to allow her to do as much as possible without compromising the sterility of the equipment or even her own safety.

When I opened the syringe packets, I let her grasp the plastic wrapper, pull it off (the needles were all capped, so this was safe for her), and put the wrapper in the trash bag. Her brow furrowed just a little.

"Are you going to give Papa a shot?" she asked.

"Not really, but I'm going to use these needles to draw out some of this saline from the bag that's hanging up there, and some heparin from this little bottle, to use in the tubes for Papa's treatment" I explained. "So he'll get the liquid, but I don't have to poke him with these needles." I wasn't sure how she'd react when we got to the part with the needles I *did* have to poke him with! At least those were attached to long clear tubing, and not instantly recognizable to her like the syringes were.

When the time came to get those out, I lifted the packet and looked questioningly at BJ, who was standing watch behind the couch. He understood my mute query: "should she see this part?" and nodded slightly. It was OK. If she was interested, it wouldn't hurt her to learn.

We opened the packet; again, I grasped the tubes within while Megan gently pulled off the plastic and disposed of it, then returned to hover at my shoulder as I sat in front of Larry and cleaned the access area over the fistula in his left upper arm with an alcohol wipe. I removed the plastic cap from the needle end of the first tube. She didn't miss a thing.

"Oh, Papa, dat's gonna hurt," she told him.

119

"Well, then, I won't watch," he assured her.

"I will!" she replied. And she did. Then afterward, with both needles successfully inserted and safely taped into place and covered with gauze pads for cushion and cleanliness, she observed seriously: "Papa, you are a very brave boy."

"Well, thank you," he told her.

"One time, I went to the doctor and had to get a shot, and I didn't even cry," she informed us. "And Mama gave me ice cream!"

That sounded like a fitting reward to us, too, and we told her so. When it was time to push the green button to start the dialysis machine, she tried her best but couldn't apply enough pressure to trigger the switch. Obviously the designers of the machine didn't want anything to start by accident. I pushed it myself, then showed her the deep red flow progressing through one of the clear plastic tubes connected to Larry's arm.

"Papa, it's taking you blood!" she sounded horrified.

"That's OK," we assured her, "it's supposed to do that." I showed her how it was going through the tubing of the cartridge in the machine and remarked on the filter getting pale pink, then pinker, and then red, and how the blood would continue to flow through the circuit of tubing to come back to Papa.

"See, here it is; it's Comin' Round the Mountain." I was trying to keep this upbeat, not wanting her to be afraid.

"Dere's a mountain?" Clearly the song I had referred to was not in her repertoire.

"Well, we can pretend the machine is the mountain. The blood goes through the machine and gets cleaned in the filter, and comes back to Papa. He doesn't lose it. He gets it back."

She was still a little skeptical, but could see that both tubes—out and in—were now fully red, and that seemed to satisfy her.

"OK," she said, but obviously with some reservation.

Then I asked her: "Megan, when you grow up, are you going to be a nurse, so you can help people like Papa who need these treatments?"

"No," she shook her head.

"Well, are you maybe going to be a doctor, and find a way to cure people so they don't have to have these treatments?"

"Yes," she nodded.

Larry's eyes twinkled, and he smiled. Time will tell.

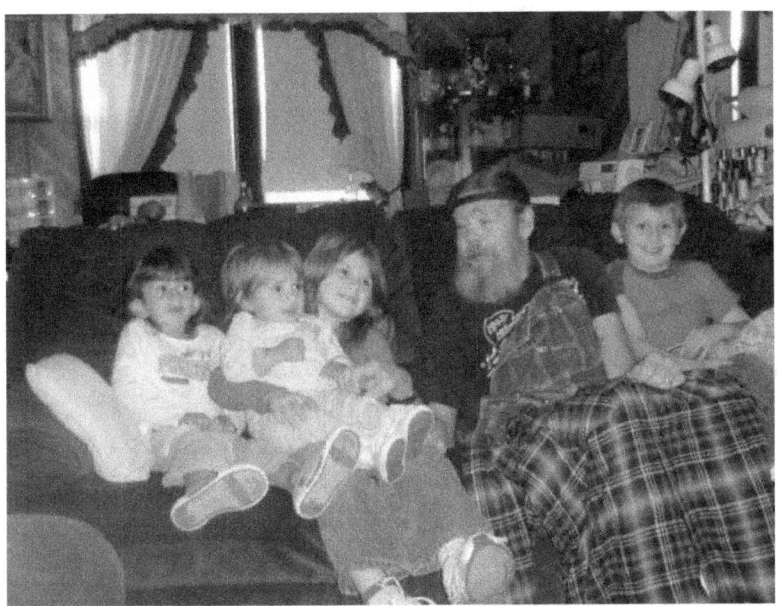

Papa and his Grandchildren

15

RUNNING ON EMPTY

In January 2010 when I was listing potentially pertinent facts and figures for the tax accountant's office, I calculated we'd spent almost $5,300 out of pocket for medical expenses between the two of us, in addition to the $3,380 I'd had set aside pre-tax from my paycheck in a Flexible Spending Account, and that we'd driven 6,120 miles for medical purposes in 2009. This mileage count was a huge decrease from 2008, when Larry began with dialysis in-center, went for training on the home-use machine, and began all the initial testing for the transplant program: That year we logged 12,562 medical miles, had more than $7,200 in after-tax medical expenses, and received reimbursement of $1,800 more in medical expenditures from my pre-tax flex account. Once more I was reminded of how much the American Kidney Fund was helping us by paying more than $3,000 a year in premiums for Larry's Medicare supplement policy.

2010 would prove lighter in the mileage department, and not quite so many appointments. Larry had laser surgery on his right eye on January 18 to correct a slight blurriness. On March 5, he underwent another endoscope procedure to receive Botox injections in the pyloric sphincter muscle, where food leaves the stomach for the duodenum. One of the side effects of long-term diabetes is often gastroparesis, a condition in which food stays in the stomach longer than it should because of partial paralysis of those muscles. Diabetes mellitus is a common cause of many types of nerve damage, and this is just one of those. The symptoms in Larry's case were indigestion, roller-coaster blood sugar readings, lack of appetite, feeling bloated, and frequent nausea. Our hope was that the Botox would help his digestive process enough to alleviate the symptoms and perhaps even allow him to eat more. Every month the blood work for the dialysis clinic and the subsequent dietician's report mentioned his lack of protein stores. But how do you bring up someone's nutrition level if they feel as though they can't eat? The printouts over the course of that year show his albumin levels in the 3.2 to 3.6 range, with a goal of 4.0 or higher, and the nurse, the dietician, the doctor, and I were all encouraging Larry to eat more protein. I tried to tempt him with various kinds of meat, nuts, cheese, etc, but the only one in the house gaining any weight was me, and I most certainly didn't need any extra.

* * *

June 30, 2010, we were back in Columbia so Larry could be measured for a new prosthesis. Dennis told us Larry's hips were not level and that this was surely contributing to the back pain. In making the new leg they'd try to correct this.

While there, Larry received a cell phone call from the transplant office; it was time to update the echo test on his heart for the team's annual review. Since we were already in town, and even in the neighborhood, we stopped by Dr. Spaedy's office. Thanks to Paula at the front desk of the Missouri Heart Center, Larry was able to have the test at 2:30 that afternoon. The follow-up letter from Dr. Spaedy dated July 26, 2010, again pronounced the results "very good. Your overall heart muscle strength remains excellent. Your valves are all working well." I hurried to fax the letter to the team at University Hospital.

The following day had already been scheduled for Larry's annual review appointments: blood draw and chest x-ray in the morning, a visit with the social worker at noon, another with the transplant nephrologist at 1 pm. When these were all complete, he made a stop by the Hanger Prosthetics office for the first fitting of his new leg.

As elated as we were over the fantastic report from the echocardiogram, it wasn't exactly what the transplant team had in mind; it had been 2 years since the cardiac stress test had been done, and they wanted a repeat of that procedure. Larry met with Dr. Spaedy on September 15 for this, even though he wasn't feeling especially good; he just wanted to get the test done and out of the way. Whether from the toxins left in his body in spite of dialysis, the effects of the dialysis itself, the back pain that was barely tolerable even with the strong pain medications, the side effects of those medications, the stomach problems from the diabetes (and the meds), or a combination of all of the above, he was only getting about 2 to 3 "good" days each week. We had no way to predict which days those would be, but just appreciated them when they occurred.

Dr. Spaedy's letter of September 20 was not as glowing as the ECG report, and indicated "some new changes compared to your test from a couple of years ago." He also wrote, "At some point we would consider rechecking the bypasses just to be sure you have not developed some significant additional blockage." The transplant team agreed with this plan, so a heart catheterization, or angiogram, was set up for October 6. Larry did pass the test, although not with flying colors, as they say; his left ventricular systolic function was at the lower end of normal. It was good enough to keep him on the transplant list, with the added precaution of meeting with a cardiologist at University Hospital on November 24. It made sense to have a heart specialist on their premises who had reviewed the file, met with the patient, and compared opinions with Dr. Spaedy. Dr. Aggarwal recommended no changes in treatment or additional tests, and sent his approval to the transplant team.

* * *

Christmas 2010 rolled around, and for the third year in a row we did not put up a Christmas tree. This was a rough thing, because we both really enjoyed seeing the tree up and all the festive feelings that come with getting it decorated and having the tiny multicolored lights on each evening. Larry and I had actually purchased a new artificial tree in November 2008, but the big cardboard box had never been opened. First there was the matter of space; the dialysis machine and all the supplies took up a lot of room. Second, the problem of time; between working full time, driving up and down the highway for medical appointments, and running dialysis treatments 5 times a week, each minute seemed to be at a premium for me. Larry was traditionally the one to put up the tree, sometimes with my help or Jennifer's, but often by himself, letting me join in for stringing the lights and hanging ornaments. But these days his back pain and the various side effects of the pain medications were limiting in the extreme. In fact, when Christmas Day arrived, I drove alone to dine at Jennifer and BJ's house. I called ahead to alert them that Larry just was not up to coming this time, knowing that the grandchildren, especially, would be disappointed not to see Papa that day.

Larry was missing out on most of the fun things in life, and the day after Christmas we talked about it in depth. To control the pain, he was using a 75-mcg fentanyl patch, plus Percocet tablets (10/325 mg), 1 or 2 at a time. Some days he could get by without the pills, but some days he watched the clock waiting for that 4th hour to expire when he could take more. Sometimes his mind was clear, but other times it was really fuzzy. He'd forget to tell me about phone calls. I couldn't tell him a joke without having to explain it afterward, which rather takes the fun out of the concept. He hadn't felt well enough to attend the funeral for his sister's husband, Ben Kuhn, earlier that month. Often Jennifer would stop by after work to visit with him, but if he was sleeping well she hated to wake him, knowing how many nights he simply couldn't sleep. If this was a day I'd been out of the house working, I'd ask him about it when I got home; he usually wasn't even aware she'd been there. We didn't know what should be done, but he agreed we should investigate further. On the 27th I called Dr. Ryan's office and talked to Sue. The first available appointment was for January 24.

"Sign him up," I told her. "Surely there's something that will help."

* * *

In the meantime, 2010's records showed that we'd driven 4,140 miles for medical reasons over the course of the year. By choosing a Medicare Part D prescription plan that cost a bit more ($77.30 per month premium), Larry had prescription coverage on generic drugs during the coverage gap (the "donut hole" they call it), and this insurance paid $3,628 on medications in 2010. After being reimbursed for $5,000 worth of medical expenses with pre-tax money from my flex account at work, our out-of-pocket figure was $3,262. Even with good insurance, quality health care isn't free.

16

A PRETTY BIG DEAL

The transplant team wanted Larry to follow-up with the gastrointestinal department again. We'd gotten a letter in December confirming that an appointment had been scheduled for January 13, 2011. When we got there, Dr. T. explained he wanted Larry to have a fasting CT scan to recheck his pancreas and liver. He would compare the new results with the previous scans for any changes. And (of course) they drew blood for the CA 19-9 test.

The scan was performed on January 24, and we were advised to see another doctor in their clinic across town for the results... in 6 weeks! While we were in the building, though, we went to the clinic office where I asked for the blood test results from the 13th. It took quite a while, but a nurse was able to print a copy of the lab report. The number next to the CA 19-9 indicator was 123; the same level he'd had in December 2008. We took this as a good sign.

* * *

The 24th was also the appointment with the neurosurgeon, Dr. Ryan. He repeated the reflex and range-of-motion tests, then ordered an MRI to check for any changes that might have taken place since the neck surgery the year before. Once more, Sue worked her magic over the phone and Larry had an MRI of his lumbar spine at 4:15 that afternoon at Boone Hospital.

Dr. Ryan called us on the 26th. The MRI showed a possible compression fracture, but rather than the lumbar spine area, it was just above this at the lower end of the thoracic region, specifically T10-T11. The images in the scan from Monday gave him just an inkling of the problem; he needed better pictures of the thoracic area to be sure. Another MRI was scheduled for the following day.

As promised, Dr. Ryan called back on Friday the 28th with the results of the second MRI. At the upper lumbar level, the L1-L2 and L3-L4 collapsed disks exhibited no change. However, vertebra T10 had completely collapsed into T11 with a 40-degree angulation, pinching Larry's spinal cord. No wonder he could barely move around! Dr. Ryan outlined the options. He could perform surgery, removing the broken pieces of backbone, using at least part of them plus some graft material to reconstruct the collapsed vertebra, and install a titanium cage, screws, and rods to hold it all in place. He anticipated Larry would be in the ICU overnight and spend 5 to 7 days in the hospital.

"It's a pretty big deal," he told me over the phone. "I would want to run it by Dr. Spaedy and Dr. Winkelmeyer, and probably divide the process into 2 separate days so we don't have to keep him under for so many hours at a time."

"And if he doesn't undergo the surgery?"

"Well, the pinching of the spinal cord would not be relieved; in fact it would soon become worse and Larry would end up in a wheelchair permanently. Frankly, I'm amazed that he can get up and walk around as much as he does." Dr. Ryan wasn't mincing words. His normal course was to take the most conservative approach possible, so I knew he wasn't recommending this surgery lightly. After I'd had a chance to discuss it with Larry, I called back to let Dr. Ryan know we wanted to go ahead. I asked him the technical name of the procedure.

"It would be a T10-T11 corpectomy with PEEK interbody cage and lateral plate; also a T10-T11 laminectomy with pedical screws and a T8-to-L1 posterior lateral fusion."

I wrote it down.

"What's PEEK?" I asked. "Is that a type of titanium?"

"No, I had thought about using titanium," Dr. Ryan explained, "but PEEK is a different type of material that works similarly and often has better results with this type of thing." He may also have told me what the letters stood for, but if he did, it was long and complicated and I didn't write it down. I've since looked it up on the Internet: polyetheretherketone.

After the standard pre-operative blood draw, EKG, chest x-ray, and one more CT scan on February 7, it was time to prepare for a week away from home. Our cell phones were both 4 years old, and technology had changed a lot in that time. Knowing I wouldn't want to lug a laptop computer around with me everywhere, but also desirous of being able to stay in touch with family and friends

127

via email, I made the leap to an iPhone, which proved to be a very valuable tool. I was even able to address a few issues at work by using it.

At 8 am on Thursday, February 10, 2011, we arrived at Boone Hospital in Columbia. Dr. Ryan (neurosurgeon) and an assisting thoracic surgeon took Larry in to surgery mid-morning and stayed there several hours. Accessing his spine through his left side, they delicately removed the broken bone fragments, sent some to the lab to be sure they were OK to reuse (they were), then recycled the pieces along with a graft from Larry's rib and a metal plate to rebuild the collapsed vertebra. They transfused 3 units of blood during the process, and then sent Larry to the Neuro ICU for the night.

My parents were there most of the day, keeping me company in the surgery waiting room, and were as relieved as I was when Dr. Ryan came out to tell us the first part of this double-barreled surgery had gone well. I stayed at the hospital that night and was allowed to rest in a recliner next to Larry's bed in the curtained ICU cubicle. Early the next morning, as Larry was just starting to wake up from the anesthetic, it was time to go back to the operating room.

Friday at 4:20 pm, Dr. Ryan reported they were done. He'd inserted two metal rods along Larry's spine, one on each side, screws from the T7 level down to L2, and bone graft material on both sides to aid in the fusion process. They'd given one more unit of blood that day, and he told me my husband would be heading back to the Neuro ICU when he left the recovery room. Dr. Ryan thought Larry might be moved to a regular room by Sunday, providing all went well.

Whether from 2 days of anesthetic in a row, the lack of dialysis for a second day, the pain medications, or a combination thereof, I could tell when they wheeled Larry out of the elevator and around the corner toward the Neuro ICU doors that he wasn't responding well. Holding his arms up above his chest, wringing his hands and sometimes flailing about, he was yelling.

"Damn it, damn it, damn it, damn it!" Over and over. Loudly.

Now, on the surface, the sentiment sounds appropriate to the

128

amount of pain he was likely in and the circumstances he'd just experienced, but having been through more than 27 years with this guy, I knew this was a unique reaction to the situation. Larry typically took a long time to come out from under anesthetic, but had never before been hostile or belligerent when he did. It was almost as if he was drunk, but I couldn't really say, as I'd rarely seen him take a drink and had never, *ever* seen him anything close to drunk. It was more than a little disconcerting. But he had been through 2 long days of major surgery, and we hoped a night's rest would have him more like himself the following day.

No such luck, though. Larry's blood sugar levels stayed stable, his oxygen saturation was fine, and he had dialysis in the afternoon, which we all hoped would help flush more of the anesthetic from his system. But he wasn't really waking up, was not opening his eyes, and was still yelling a lot, just as he had all night. They'd moved him from the curtained cubicle to a glass-walled room at the edge because his frequent, loud calling was a disturbance to other patients. And although he did cough three separate times at my request, and even move each of his legs a little bit when I asked him to, Larry didn't respond to these same questions from Dr. Ryan, and of course the doctor didn't happen to be in the room when Larry did those things for me. So in essence, "it never happened," which I understand. If the surgeon didn't witness the occurrence, how can he possibly put it in the record?

Sunday February 13th held more of the same, and the care staff was getting worried. At 10 am they wheeled Larry down to radiology for a CT scan and an MRI. They didn't tell me what they were looking for, exactly, but my impression was they were checking to see if Larry had suffered a stroke. He definitely should have been awake by now; it was more than 40 hours post-surgery. I hadn't been scared until then, but the potential ramifications shook me. I called my sister Janice and she talked with me, calm and soothing.

The tests came out OK, and Dr. Ryan decided to switch Larry's pain meds from the morphine IV drip to liquid Percocet through a tube, with morphine boluses available if needed. Finally at 4 pm Larry opened his eyes just a few times, and flexed his right knee once. He also answered a couple of questions for a nurse ("yes" and "no" sort of stuff), but was still agitated, flailing his arms and calling out. They put padded mittens on his hands, strapped at the wrists with Velcro tabs, to keep him from pulling loose the various tubes attached to his body. It was a rough day. Dr. Ryan was very serious as he told me, "We don't always get the outcome we hope for, and this may be one of those times." I think he wanted to believe things would improve, but by this point was afraid of getting his hopes up... or mine.

Monday was Valentine's Day, but my sweetheart was in no mood for hearts or flowers. The extreme agitation continued, with the waving of arms, beating his hands against the pillows we placed on his torso to protect him from himself, and still more yelling. When I arrived that morning from the hotel room I'd taken, a nurse was administering a bolus of morphine. I politely but firmly requested NO MORE MORPHINE, and the doctors agreed to try other avenues for pain control. The chest tube for drainage was removed, Larry was taken to the hospital's dialysis clinic for his treatment, and finally that afternoon he moved his legs for Dr. Ryan!

The yelling was diminishing somewhat, and changed from "no, no, no, no, no" to "Owwwwww" that afternoon.

"Where do you hurt?" I asked him.

"I don't know," he replied.

At least it was an answer!

Once the morphine began making its way out of Larry's system, he began making some progress. Tuesday the 15th he made short statements: "I need a drink" and "That's enough." He also drank from a straw: ice water, grape juice, chicken broth, tea, and diet cola. Twice he even swallowed a pill with the liquid. The doctor removed the drain from his back, but wrote orders to have a PICC line and a Corpak (feeding tube) put in. The first one was for IV-type medications and extended from his right arm to an artery in his chest; the second went through his nose down to his stomach and would be used to give him other liquid medications and nutritional supplements. Even though he was picking up liquids through the straw, he'd been without food for almost a week, and his body would have a hard time healing from the surgery without adequate food intake.

On Wednesday at 6 pm Larry was finally moved out of the ICU and into a regular hospital room. He'd had dialysis that day and drunk a bottle of Ensure at breakfast and lunchtime, but was still very sleepy, rather grumpy, and somewhat uncooperative. That last trait continued on into the next day, when it became supplemented by "rude" as I tried to comb all the snarls out of his hair. And when I turned my attention to speak to the nurse for a moment, she and I were both surprised when we glanced back at Larry to witness him pulling the Corpak line out of his nose. We must've both made exclamations of some sort because he just sort of froze, sitting there with his hand in the air and an expression on his face that said, "What did I do?" The fact was, he really didn't know what he was doing. The pain medications had him so loopy he simply couldn't comprehend what was going on, and weeks later when we talked about those days, he had no clear memory of them. For the most part, that was probably a good thing.

It wasn't until Saturday February 19—9 days after the initial surgery—that Larry was able to have solid food. He'd had a terribly bad dream the night before, and his big goal that day was trying to convince me to get him *out* of there, immediately! As I explained that he wasn't well enough to leave yet, he became convinced I was part of a conspiracy to hold him against his will. When his brother called my cell phone, I put it on speaker for Larry to be able to talk to him, too… whereupon he begged Tom to come rescue him. Later in the day sister Susan and our niece Rebekah came to visit. They were greeted warmly, right up to the time they had to deny his request to "get me OUT of here, NOW!" At least I wasn't alone on the Bad Guy List. Poor Larry!

"Do your parents know you're keeping me here like this?" he asked me at some point that day. Geez! Talk about a guilt trip.

The day wasn't all bad, though. I enjoyed the visit with Susan and Rebekah, and when the physical therapist came to the room to work with Larry, he sat up on the side of the bed for a bit and did about 50% of the work of getting himself there, the therapist told me. The day before, he'd done about 25% of the effort, so this was definite progress.

The next day he sat up in a recliner and then a wheelchair for about an hour, and on Monday he worked with the physical therapists again on sitting up and finally on standing for a couple of minutes. Dr. Ryan talked to us about Larry's release from the hospital, explaining that he was too weak to go straight home, but his recovery could continue in a skilled nursing facility where physical therapists would work with him on a daily basis to improve his strength, balance, and motor skills until he was strong enough to be safe at home. He estimated this might take as little as a couple of weeks, but probably more like a month. A social worker from the hospital was assigned to help locate a facility with the level of care he would require plus the ability to transport Larry to and from his dialysis treatments three times a week.

The incisions in Larry's back had been closed with staples; I think I counted 97 of them. They were very close together and looked like two zippers in an upside-down Y-shape down his spine and off to the left. The staples came out on Tuesday, February 22. Dr. Ryan had cautioned that this surgery would be a "pretty big deal", and he was right. What we couldn't know at that point was that the "big deal" wasn't over yet. The recovery phase was just beginning.

17
A ROUGH RECUPERATION

It took a few days to get everything coordinated for the move, but on Monday, February 28, Larry arrived by ambulance at Clinton Healthcare and Rehabilitation center, about 25 miles from home. The facility in our little town of Windsor would have been more convenient for me to visit each day after work, but they weren't set up for transporting patients to dialysis. The nearest dialysis clinic was in Clinton, and the care center chosen had a van with a wheelchair lift that would take Larry to and from the clinic three times a week for his treatments. The nurses at the care center would be responsible for providing his medications and keeping track of his blood sugar readings, and an on-site physical therapist would work with Larry while he recovered to help him regain his strength and balance.

The first full day was spent regrouping from the transfer, but on Wednesday in therapy Larry walked 8 steps. That earned an underline, an exclamation point, and a smiley face in my steno pad of notes. Thursday he walked 16 steps and seemed on the right track for making progress until about 8 pm, when one of the nurses called me at home.

"Larry's lungs sound raspy to me this evening, and he's coughing up some nasty-looking stuff" she reported. "We're going to get him over to the emergency room for a chest x-ray."

I met him at the Golden Valley Medical Center ER, where the doctor on call diagnosed pneumonia in both lungs and prescribed a strong antibiotic along with breathing treatments. Whether this was from a bacteria picked up in Columbia or from all the days of being flat on his back and basically out of it after the surgery was unclear, but most likely the latter. The treatment worked, but it set Larry back in the recovery process. He felt awful, and over the next few days he didn't want to cooperate with the therapists who were trying to help him get better. To be fair, his brain function was still pretty fuzzy from the after-effects of the surgery and (I believe) the morphine reaction; each day when I visited we'd play a little quiz game, with me asking him annoying questions like "What day is this?" "What town are we in now?" and "What are the names of our grandchildren?" Some days were better than others, and Larry's memory was improving with time. Still, he seemed to be sinking into a depression and remained convinced that I could take him home if I just *wanted* to.

Jennifer and BJ both had jobs in Clinton and were stopping by to see him as often as possible, she in the morning and he in the late afternoon. It was a man-to-man visit from his son-in-law that really helped Larry to turn the corner. BJ went by for a visit and helped Larry into the wheelchair parked beside the bed. He pushed the chair outside into the fresh air and sunshine of mid-March. They sat in a gazebo near the building where they could watch the busy traffic on one of the main streets of Clinton. BJ knew it was time for some frank talk about the way things were going. He and Jennifer and the kids had been praying for Larry's continued healing from the physical part of the ordeal, but it was apparent the mental/emotional part of the equation needed help, too.

"Dad, you know we care about you. We all—Jenny, me, the kids, Mom—we all want to see you get better. We want to see you come home. We want you to be safe when you get there, to be able to get up and walk to the kitchen or the bathroom or out onto the front porch with the walker or a cane or whatever. Mom's been busy moving things around so you'll have plenty of room for the walker and nothing in the way that would trip you. She's even bought you a new recliner that's really comfortable and should feel good to your back. But you have to make an effort here. The therapists are willing to work with you and help you regain your strength, but they can't make you do the exercises. You have to decide if you want to come home enough to work for it. Ever since we met you've told me you're not a quitter. We're here for you, but you need to try."

For BJ, it was one of the longest uninterrupted talks he'd ever delivered. It felt just a little chancy, somehow, giving advice to his father-in-law, but he felt strongly that these were the words Larry needed at the time. Apparently he was right. The next day when I arrived to visit, Larry was sitting up in the wheelchair and ready to move around. He'd been to the dining room for all his meals that day and had made more progress in physical therapy. I complimented him on his demeanor and his positive outlook, and he told me that BJ had had a talk with him the day before.

"I think it really helped me," Larry told me. "I needed to hear what he said. I knew those things, but I just needed to hear them. And I guess I needed to hear them from him."

His smile was sincere, and there was a light in my husband's eyes again that had been missing lately.

"He's a good man, isn't he?" Larry said, referring to BJ.

"Yes, Darlin'," I agreed, "he's a very good man."

*   *   *

Larry's progress in physical therapy wasn't instantaneous, but it was sure and steady, albeit slow. By the time we went back to Columbia on March 28 for x-rays at the hospital and the post-surgical visit with Dr. Ryan across the street, Larry was using a walker and getting around fairly well. He didn't try to walk very far at a time, and certainly didn't move fast, but at least he was moving! The doctor pronounced Larry fit to come home, and wrote orders for physical therapists to come to the house and work with him three times each week for the next month. We kept a wheelchair on hand "just in case" but didn't need to use it. Having a ramp from the sidewalk up to the back door made it easier for Larry to navigate with the walker, and later with a cane, and at the end of the sidewalk where it sloped downward to the driveway and the surface was rocky and uneven, we were really glad to have the raised platform a friend had built so Larry would have a level surface about the same height as the running boards on the old Suburban for getting into and out of the vehicle. We hired that same friend to expand the bathroom on the ground floor of our house to include a walk-in shower with a seat and hand rails for safety.

With Larry's back on the mend, it was time to look into his status on the transplant list. He'd been categorized as "inactive" back in January when it was clear he would be going in for back surgery. This meant he continued to accumulate days on The List, but even if a match came up, he was unavailable for transplant surgery. I called the transplant nurse coordinator and found out that because of the severity of the surgery and the fact that metal hardware was implanted, Larry would remain "inactive" for at least 6 months after the operation, to give his body plenty of time to heal and to be sure no infections were lurking around in his system. Although somewhat disappointing, the news made sense. We were, after all, trying to improve his health, not put him at greater risk.

The 6-month post-surgery date was August 11, 2011, and true to their word, the transplant team began gearing up on Larry's behalf a couple weeks ahead of that with the information that the annual tests were due, and to start things off with a cardiac stress test on August 8. Dr. Spaedy's letter this time was more encouraging, noting the test results were slightly improved from those of 2010. The following day involved blood work, a chest x-ray, and visits with the nephrologist, the nurse coordinator, and the social worker at University Hospital.

The next step was August 19, when we met with a doctor in the Digestive Health clinic. He informed us the CT scan that had been performed back in January showed no sign of the lesions on Larry's liver that had appeared in the previous tests, but that his pancreatic duct was still dilated. Overall, during the course of the three years of testing, he saw improvement in the liver/pancreas areas, but just to be sure everything was okay, he wanted to schedule another endoscopic ultrasound (EUS). Knowing that a kidney transplant would immediately put Larry on a regimen of immune-suppressant drugs to keep him from rejecting the organ, the doctor reminded us that an abundance of caution was in order to verify that there were no underlying cancer cells brewing in his body.

The EUS procedure was conducted on Thursday, September 1, and the report showed that everything appeared very similar to the same test that had been done 3 years earlier. A lab report on the biopsy samples was issued on September 8, with the good news: "negative for malignancy or adenoma" and "no evidence of cancer or infection." Still, we had to attend a follow-up visit with the doctor on September 23 to hear him say, "I see no reason that you should not be active again on the kidney list."

Boy, were we ever glad to hear those words! Just to get the ball rolling, they drew blood that day for the monthly cross-match supply. And on Friday, October 7, Larry received the phone call that he was once again "active" on the waiting list for a kidney. By this time he had been on dialysis more than three and a half years. After all the testing, surgery, retesting, more surgery, and retesting yet again, we were *so* ready for a kidney transplant!

18

WE ARRIVE AT KIDNEYILLE

Sunday, October 9, 2011

The first call came about 12:15 am, after we'd both been asleep about 2 hours, which was against House Rules. Back when our daughter was in junior high and the phone calls all seemed to be for her, I'd had to lay down the law.

"If this phone rings after 9 pm," I'd told her, "it means someone has died... or someone is about to."

Not a very nice way to say "no calls after 9 pm," but effective. She needed sleep for school, I needed sleep for work, and our nerves didn't need to jump at the startle of a late-night phone ringing.

That being said... when you're waiting for a kidney, that same phone could ring at any hour with news of hope and we wouldn't mind a bit. During the fall of 2010 we'd had one such call from Andrew Webb, RN, one of the coordinators with the transplant team. He'd telephoned to let us know they had an offer of a kidney from an Iowa donor, and that Larry was number 6 in line. Three people in Iowa would be tested first and then three people in Missouri, as potential recipients.

He had questions for Larry:

- Was he feeling well?

- Did he have any fever now, or within the last couple of weeks?

- When had he last dialyzed?

- Did he have any open wounds?

- Had he taken any antibiotics within the past several weeks?

- Did he take any blood thinners, and if so, when was the most recent dose?

- When did he last eat?

He then explained that they hadn't yet seen the donor's kidney and so had no idea if it was viable for transplant; this call was just a "yellow alert" for us and a marshaling of possible recipients. The Iowa folks would be in line ahead of the Missouri folks because of the location of the donor. Andrew promised to call back when he knew more, and he fulfilled that promise: "No go." Once the doctors in Iowa saw the kidney they could tell it would not be good for transplant. They were sorry. We were, too, but it had seemed Larry's chances at this particular organ were slim anyway.

"It's OK," we told Andrew over the phone. "We appreciate the family's willingness to offer, and your call to give us a heads-up."

Andrew advised that it is not uncommon to receive several such calls of potential donors before the day came that Larry might actually receive a kidney.

And now here was the second call, just 36 hours after we'd heard Larry had gone "active" on the list again. Andrew asked Larry the same questions. This time, however, Larry was #3 in line, there were two potential kidneys on offer, and they were right here in Missouri. If either of the patients ahead of Larry on the list did not "mix," then he would move up to #2. If both kidneys were viable... well, you get the idea.

"When will the lab results be in on the cross-match?" I asked.

"Probably around 6 or 7 am," Andrew replied, "and I'll let you know when I hear."

Wow.

We were stunned.

Could this be IT? Had the day we'd been hoping for finally arrived?

"No way can I go back to sleep now!" I told Larry after the call was finished and we'd both taken a couple of deep breaths. "Guess I'll go see what I can get done at my desk, just in case."

I sat in my office chair and fired up the company laptop.

Thought about the call.

Went back to the living room, knelt in front of Larry.

"We need to pray for that family."

He agreed.

139

We did.

Somehow Larry was able to lean back in his recliner and go back to sleep.

* * *

There were several files at my desk earmarked for Monday's workday, and I was able to get some work done in the still of the night.

Albert, my dog, stretched out on his cushion by the bookshelf, and Jack, the three-legged cat, stayed close to me on the desk, on the top of my chair's backrest, or (when he could finagle it) on me. It's a fact that I was instrumental in snatching Jack back from the Jaws of Death twice in his first 18 months of life, and he doesn't show any signs of forgetting that. Sticks to me like glue. Like white on rice. Like stink on... well, you get my meaning.

By 6 am I was wearing down, getting sleepy again. I relaxed with a little time on "www.sporcle.com", the website of "mentally stimulating diversions":

"100 most common British surnames"
"100 most used words in American English"
"Name the Presidents"
"Popular Baby Boy Names of the 1920s"
"Countries of the World"

. . . and stuff like that. I call them "mental health moments," which may be a simple attempt to justify blowing time on computer games; but then again, it can't hurt to exercise the ol' noodle now and then, can it? (Did I mention I majored in Procrastination in college?) Maybe I thought that actually having everything ready to go out the door would "jinx" our chances?

7 am and no further phone call. I checked the phone—yes, we had a dial tone. (Yawn) "Larry, I'm gonna take a nap."

"OK," and he was back to sleep.

* * *

9:30 am. Andrew's second call.

"The lab results came back, and Larry, you are now in the #2 slot. We'd like you to come on over to the hospital and get admitted and prepped for surgery."

"WOW!"

That was the only word either of us could think of.

"Have you eaten anything today?" Andrew asked.

"No."

"OK, good. Come on over and tell them you are to be admitted for surgery. Since it's Sunday there may not be anyone at the Admissions desk, so just go on down the hall to the ER and they'll let us know you're here."

"Um, Andrew?" I hesitated, "I still need to do some things around here to get our stuff together, make arrangements for being gone, you know... "

"OK, when do you think you might arrive?"

(Quick calculations, mental checklists)

"Probably no sooner than 1 pm."

"That's fine; we'll see you this afternoon."

Somewhere in there was also a statement that the donor had not yet been to surgery, so they'd not actually confirmed visually that two viable kidneys would be available for transplant. So we were excited, but still cognizant of the possibility that this could all end up as a dress rehearsal of sorts and that we could easily get to Columbia, only to be sent back home with a "Sorry—maybe another day." Is that why I didn't have our things together when Andrew called back? Was it the fear that counting on something too much might "jinx" it and pop the bubble of hope? Who knows?

But the sense of urgency prevailed now for sure.

Larry got into the shower.

I called our daughter Jennifer to request that she or BJ stop by the house each day to check on things, bring in the mail, feed the multitude of critters. Told her about the call and what was happening. Told her if things went as planned we'd probably be in Columbia at least a week. Since Jennifer works nights (and Sunday night is the start of her workweek), BJ works days, and three of their four children were already in school, I did not expect them to make this trip with us.

"Sure." she replied. But she sounded a little quiet.

141

"Aren't you excited?" I asked.

"Yeah... anxious," she admitted.

"Well, babe, just remember who's in control, right?"

"I know, God's in control."

"It'll be OK, whatever happens." I told her.

"I know, I just..."

"I know. We love you bunches, and thanks for looking after things."

"You're welcome. Let me know, OK?"

"I will. Promise."

Then I called my parents and spoke with Mother. A quick explanation, just wanted them to know. We agreed she could let my siblings know, but at this point the news didn't need to go any further.

"It may turn out to be a dry run," Mother said. "But at least it's a chance."

Then I took a quick survey around the house. What *had* to be done, and what could wait?

I ran a load of laundry, packed a bag for me and one for Larry, and cleaned out and then filled food and water bowls in the outdoor kennel for Albert.

Then I fed the cats in the house, those outside on the porch, and those up in the pigeon loft/workshop. I checked the feed and water for the pigeons, the chickens, and guineas. The horses had grass in the pasture and water in the pond and from two automatic waterers, so they would be fine.

I changed the message on my desk phone to route business calls to my boss, sent a text message to that boss's cell phone, and set the automated reply feature on my office email account to indicate "out of office"—but didn't know what end date to set. I started with a week.

Then I gathered things to do while away: an audio book on mp3; headphones; another book on the new Kindle I'd received for my birthday; an actual book (!); crochet pattern, hook, and yarn for the afghan I'd started for Luke's birthday; the steno pad with notes I'd been keeping on Larry's medical issues the past 3+ years; a legal pad for "whatever" (as it turned out, I started writing this book on that pad); and Larry's list of current medications/medical history.

Finally I made sure the coffee pot was off, walked Albert one more time, and tried to assure him we'd be back and that Jennifer would be coming by to look after him. Then I put him in his kennel with a newly unwrapped ham bone from the store. Geez, all this was taking too long, *why* had I frittered away time on the computer in the wee hours of the morning?!

Finally, everything we thought we might need was loaded into the old white Suburban, and we were both buckled in, Larry with his pillows but without his customary glass of tea or can of soda, since they'd told him no food or drink.

"We're off!" I said, as we started down the driveway.

"Like a herd of turtles," Larry filled in.

We shared a smile.

* * *

So it wasn't 1 pm but 2:30 by the time we arrived in Columbia, found a parking spot, figured out just how much stuff we ought to carry in without looking like we were *moving* in, and made our way to the other end of the hospital to find the ER. We checked in with the lady at the desk and took a seat in the waiting room, where we were soon joined by my parents. They hadn't told me they would be making the 2-hour drive to Columbia, but it surprised neither of us; over the years, my folks had made many such trips to sit and visit with us at various hospitals. They'd entertained me with countless stories, jokes, anecdotes from my childhood, their childhoods, family vacations, etc. My dad and Larry would talk about motorcycles, or how something was built, or something from the science or nature or history channels on TV. Mother's family is a tight-knit but large clan, and there's always news of one cousin or another, and of course the grandchildren are always a favorite topic.

Finally a room was ready, and we accompanied Larry upstairs to the room where he'd wait for whatever the next steps might be. Of course, one of the first things they wanted was a blood sample. This time we were lucky and the technician was able to get the job done on her first try. Remember, Larry had had nothing to eat or drink since the evening before, and now it's mid-to-late afternoon. His veins weren't always what you'd call cooperative with this procedure, and lack of liquid intake didn't help, so we were grateful for her expertise.

Then began the parade of doctors. A kidney transplant team consists of several specialists:

- A nephrologist, who oversees how the kidney is performing

- The surgeon who actually does the transplant

- An anesthesiologist, who keeps the patient asleep for the procedure

- A urologist, who tends to bladder function

- A social worker

- A dietician

- A nurse coordinator who helps monitor medications and doctor visits

- The hospital chaplain

- And, for diabetics, an endocrinologist, who tries to keep the patient's blood sugars stable

And, since this was a teaching hospital, each of the specialists above might have two or three (maybe even four) students or less experienced doctors at various levels of their training who come in to ask questions and review the case before the actual doctor makes his or her way onto the scene. Almost all of these folks ask many of the same questions, but not (of course) at the same time. It would be easier, wouldn't it, if they'd just all sit down at a long table or in a tiered box like a jury, and put the patient on the witness stand where they could all hear the answers simultaneously? But it doesn't work that way. After about the third or fourth almost identical set of questions, Larry was getting a little cranky.

As a caregiver, it's difficult to know exactly when it's OK to run interference and jump in with answers and when it's time to back off and just observe. I could tell pretty quickly when my husband was getting prickly, and usually had a decent idea of why. I'd figured out one tool that could sometimes be a shortcut through some of this: a one-page document—which I referred to as The Document—that I had created on the laptop at home, listing Larry's name and date of birth in the upper corner, his current medications (along with am and/or pm dosage) on the top half, and a brief chronological list of his medical history (surgeries and important diagnostic events). Any time a medication was changed or a new surgery performed, I just amended The Document on the computer. A couple of times I had to change the page borders and the font style or size to keep all this to one page! But I tried to keep a current one with us at all times, and before this trip I had printed 4 copies to bring along. And as a follow-up to the ordeal of the previous winter, it was now plainly marked "Morphine Intolerant."

Please understand, having this gun in your arsenal won't prevent that friendly barrage of questions. Even providing this to the nurse at check-in and asking that it be placed in the file for all to see won't circumvent the repetition that comes from having all these cooks and one patient as the 'stew.' When the doctor/intern/whoever would come in and introduce themselves to Larry and then begin the quiz, if it seemed like my page of information would help summarize things for them, I'd reach into my nearby canvas tote bag, withdraw a copy of The Document, and politely ask if they'd seen this, or might they like a copy? Without fail, he or she would give The Document at least a quick perusal, perhaps offer a comment or pose a question for clarity, and either ask to make a copy for their own file or accept the extra I offered. Whether they kept them in a file, put them in the trash, or what, I have no way to know. They all, however, seemed to appreciate the synopsis, and it appeared to help ease the tension for Larry once they'd had a glance at the list of things he'd been through.

* * *

Mother recalls that one of the doctors—the anesthesiologist, probably—enumerated the possible risks associated with the surgery.

"Things that could happen during or after the procedure: you

145

could have a heart attack; you could develop a blood clot; you could get an infection; you could have a stroke; you could die. Now, knowing those things, do you still want to proceed with this?"

Larry had a slight, peaceful smile.

"Yes."

* * *

The typical pre-op routine of blood draw for lab tests, chest x-ray, EKG, and setting up an IV were completed. It wasn't until about 8 pm that we received word the surgery would not be taking place that night. By this point, Larry hadn't eaten anything in almost 24 hours and I asked if he might be allowed to have a light supper. The doctors agreed to this request, and Larry was glad to have a sandwich, some fruit, and some milk. At this point some patients might get nervous or worried, but this guy was taking everything in stride with equanimity, as usual. He even slept pretty well that night, in spite of not being in his own environment. The following day seemed to start off slowly also, but finally in the early afternoon they moved Larry to pre-op and he was visited (again) by that long string of doctors, with the actual transplant surgeon being one of the last to come by. It felt a little weird to ask, but I had to know: Had he actually seen the kidney yet?

"Yes, it's here, and I have seen it, and it looks just great!" he assured us. We also learned the donor was about 20 years younger than Larry, and the creatinine reading on this donated kidney was 0.4, which is fantastic.

The transplant surgery began shortly after 3 pm and was over by 9 pm. Larry weathered it well and was moved to the CICU (Cardiac Intensive Care Unit) about 11 pm. I wondered aloud if this placement was specific to Larry due to his prior bypass surgery, and learned that being in the CICU is a normal first step after receiving a kidney transplant. The team in this unit was very impressive and highly attentive to providing the best possible care.

On Tuesday, October 11, Larry was allowed a clear liquid diet. The kidney was already working, and the fluid output was carefully measured and recorded. Toward evening Larry was helped to sit up in a chair for about an hour. Another session in the

146

chair took place on Wednesday, but Larry slept through most of it. His blood glucose was holding steady, the incision looked good, and the drain had been taken out, but his oxygen saturation wasn't as high as it should be, with readings of only 86% to 90%. A chest x-ray that afternoon led to a diagnosis of pneumonia in his left lung, and IV antibiotics were started. One of the nurses told me the pulmonary (lung) specialist had ordered that Larry be sedated and intubated again so the ventilator could help him breathe for 2 to 3 days while the antibiotics worked on the pneumonia. There was logic in the statement, but I could tell from the nurse's face this might not be a good sign. At barely 48 hours after transplant, being put onto a ventilator seemed like going backward instead of forward. Cultures were taken to help diagnose exactly what type of infection he had and whether or not it was invading his bloodstream.

The next day Larry had no fever and the chest x-rays looked a bit improved. By 3 pm he was breathing easier and at 4 pm they once again took him off the ventilator. Without the sedatives, his responses were good and he began drinking fluid through a straw again. His creatinine level was 3.9, and the next day it was 3.46. These numbers were lower than we'd seen in a long time, and each time the tests were run that crucial indicator of kidney function got better and better. It was now October 14, our daughter's birthday, but her dad and I were the ones who felt like we'd truly received a gift.

19

OK TO GO

Over the next several days, Larry's creatinine levels continued to plummet: 3.04 on Saturday, 2.45 on Sunday, 2.07 on Monday, 1.67 on Tuesday, and 1.52 on Wednesday, then creeping down to 1.23 by Sunday the 23rd. This kidney was definitely working! And on Monday the 17th—exactly 1 week after the transplant—Larry was able to work with the physical therapists enough to put on his prosthetic leg, stand up from a chair to a walker, and take several steps. To celebrate this progress he was moved out of CICU and into a regular room that evening.

To say that he was feeling *good*, however, would be stretching the truth. Larry did have some pain at the incision site, though even with the surgical staples that wasn't the spot that bothered him the most. Typical of the days after any surgery, his digestive system was having to wake up again, and his tummy was frequently upset. Some days he had a good appetite, but other days he simply didn't want to eat. We'd fought this battle before, and knew it could be a difficult balance between pain medications and active (but not overactive!) digestion. Still, by Wednesday, October 19, Larry was able to eat breakfast and lunch, and my steno pad notes indicate he walked about 60 feet that afternoon using a walker and with a physical therapist close by in case he required any help. After that Larry sat in a chair for a couple of hours, staying awake and watching TV. He even managed to eat some supper. Things were looking up, and even his blood sugar readings seemed to be holding more stable than ever.

Over the next few days, Larry continued to work with physical therapy, raising himself up from either the bed or a chair and walking increasingly longer distances up and down the hallways. The weather outside was pleasant, and he enjoyed a few wheelchair rides outside into the sunshine of mid-October. He talked to some family members on the phone and was so much clearer headed than he had been after the back surgery the previous

February. One day he saw me writing on my yellow legal pad and asked what it was; I told him I had started this book, and read to him what I'd put down so far. I asked him for details on some of the episodes of his life from before we'd met, and we both had fun with the reminiscing that brought on.

Monday, October 24, was the day he'd been waiting for all weekend. The doctors had told him on Friday that he would likely get to go home on Monday, and Larry was anxious to do just that. He had been 2 weeks at the hospital, and we were both looking forward to being back in our own environment. With good lab reports, a big sack of medications, and a list of instructions, we were finally packed up into the Suburban about 5:30 pm, arriving at the farm a couple of hours later. BJ was here to help Larry make the transfer out of the truck and up the ramp into the house. The 90-mile ride home had taken a toll, and Larry was in a lot of pain from a very swollen area of highly tender, delicate skin. It was in a private location he did not wish to discuss, but at my insistence we'd had a doctor inspect the region one more time before leaving the hospital, and were told this was "typical," to use cold packs to help relieve the symptoms, and that within a couple of weeks this would subside.

The night was horrendous. Larry's stomach was highly upset, and he developed explosive diarrhea. He moaned or cried out in pain most of the time, and we did not sleep. His breathing became more like panting. The thermometer showed no fever, but he told me he felt hot and needed air. Sometime after 4 am I told him we needed help, and called 911. When the paramedics arrived, Larry's blood pressure was 110 over 68, and his pulse was 115. They immediately administered oxygen and loaded him up for the nearest ER, in Sedalia. From there the doctors would contact the team at University Hospital for further instruction.

Not having had time yet to unpack our things from the trip to Columbia 2 weeks earlier, I grabbed a few items (including the new medicines and the accompanying list) and drove to Bothwell Hospital in Sedalia. Larry was calmer, breathing better with the oxygen assistance they were giving him, and asking for something to drink. I was allowed to give him a little crushed ice from a

149

spoon and was doing that when suddenly he stopped responding, the monitor near the bed began beeping, and the nurse and doctor nearby both sprang into action. Larry's blood pressure was dropping, and doing so rapidly. They were already infusing saline as quickly as it would go through the IV they'd started before I got there. Something was drastically wrong. The doctor lowered the head of the bed and called for "the cart." I began backing toward the door, not wanting to leave, but conscious of not wanting to get in the way of medical professionals trying to do their jobs.

As I exited the cubicle, two ladies from an office joined me and walked me to the otherwise-empty waiting room outside the double doors to the Emergency Room. I heard the announcement over the speaker system "CODE BLUE." It seemed surreal. The ladies asked me if we had family nearby; I explained that our daughter was probably already asleep after her night shift, our son-in-law was at work, and all our other family was more than 100 miles away. They gently urged me to call Jennifer. As it turned out she was still awake, but had stopped to talk to BJ's Aunt Alice and Uncle Bill, who kept little Amarillo during the day while her mama was sleeping and her daddy was at work. Their house is less than 2 miles from BJ and Jennifer's, but either her cell phone wasn't getting any signal there or else it was in the truck and she wasn't. I called the concrete company in Clinton and talked to BJ. He raced to pick up his wife and bring her to Sedalia. In the meantime, my good friend Peggy Richwine had arrived to sit with me and wait for news. I used my phone to send an email to our parents and siblings, letting them know where we were and why. "We are at ER in Sedalia. Called ambulance early am as Larry was not breathing well. White count very low, possible infection. Blood pressure very low. Trying to stabilize and fly back to Columbia."

Finally at almost noon a doctor came out to see us. Larry was in the ICU. He apparently had an infection and had gone into acute respiratory failure. The word "sepsis" was in there somewhere. They were working to stabilize him for transfer back to Columbia and had been on the phone with the doctors there. Broad-spectrum antibiotics were being administered to combat the infection, and lab tests had been started in an attempt to pinpoint the type of infection so they'd know what might be the best way to combat this invader.

I sent a second brief email to immediate family: "Still in Sedalia. Moved to ICU. Still trying to stabilize blood pressure. Breathing tube in, on ventilator." And about 35 minutes after that: "Diagnosis acute respiratory failure, sepsis, and neutropenia. They are trying to get a helicopter for the transfer back to Columbia."

We were allowed to go into the ICU and visit with Larry, who was conscious, but irritated with the breathing tube for the ventilator. He tried to talk, but the tube was in the way. Jennifer understood that he didn't want that tube in his mouth and down his throat. She spoke sweetly but firmly that it was there to help him breathe and he needed to cooperate with the team trying to help him. The doctor had told us they were reluctant to use a sedative since it could lower Larry's blood pressure even more; it was dangerously low already, and they were doing everything possible to counteract that.

The winds were very strong that day… so strong that it made flying a medical helicopter perilous. The doctor told us they'd asked for Air Evac for Larry, but both the smaller and the larger, heavier helicopters were grounded due to the winds. By midafternoon they agreed that Larry was stable enough to travel the 65 miles by ambulance. Jennifer wasn't sure whether to go with me or to return home; BJ wanted to let her make her own decision, but felt strongly she should be with us in Columbia. Pulling her aside, he leveled with her: Things looked very serious, and while we hoped and prayed for the antibiotics and blood pressure medications to work, and he knew her dad had beaten the odds many times when medical professionals didn't necessarily think he would, this time might be different. And if it was, and this was "it," her daddy would need her permission to go.

So while BJ went home to be with the kids, Jennifer and I quickly grabbed a few items from the house and drove back to University Hospital in Columbia. Larry was in the Med-Neuro ICU and had yet another great team of folks doing everything in their power to help. The doctor did not sugarcoat what he had to tell us: Larry was now in severe septic shock, with multiple system organ failure. The new kidney was no longer working, his lungs had failed, his central nervous system was affected, and his blood pressure remained dangerously low (88/52) due to metabolic acidosis. The next 24 to 48 hours were critical. They were administering antibiotics and blood pressure medications, and a light sedative to keep Larry relaxed enough not to fight the ventilator. The prognosis was not good.

There wasn't much cell phone signal in the ICU, but the Internet access for my phone was working. I sent a message to our parents and siblings, and this time I included the extended family and the friends who'd been getting all the daily "good news" updates since the kidney transplant, advising them of what we'd just been told. It was 6 pm.

We were able to visit with Larry a little while, and he was able to open his eyes now and then. He appeared to be resting comfortably, though, and dozed off frequently. When I told him that Jennifer and I would go back to the nearby hotel where I'd spent my nights during the previous couple of weeks so we could rest for a bit, he nodded his agreement. I kissed his forehead and told him, "I love you!"

"Love you," he mouthed around the vent tube.

* * *

One of the nurses had written our cell phone numbers on the note board in Larry's room, and I called her from the hotel at 9:30 pm to provide the phone number and our room number there. Things were about the same, she told me; Larry's blood pressure was about 90/60, and they were transfusing a couple of units of blood.

Jennifer had fallen asleep as soon as her head hit the pillow, but it was a short night. The phone rang at 1:40 am, and one of the doctors we'd met in the ICU told me there was no sign of improvement in Larry's condition. In fact, she told me gently, "Things are looking pretty bad here." She felt we should return to the hospital. I roused Jennifer and tried hard to obey the traffic laws for the few miles we had to travel.

The medical team members were sober as one of the doctors

explained the situation to us. The infection was the result of gram-negative bacteria, which is very difficult to counteract. The normal early symptoms of an infection may have been masked by some of the medications Larry was taking because of the transplant, and now his blood pressure was only 66/61. With 100% airflow, his oxygen saturation levels were only 88% at best. The machines were doing all the work. It was only a matter of time, he said. Larry's body was shutting down.

Jennifer and I sat with him, each holding one of his hands. Larry was sleeping or perhaps comatose; he wasn't opening his eyes, and didn't squeeze our hands or respond in any way. It was very quiet as the various members of the medical team softly came and went from their workstation right outside the door of the glass-walled room. Finally, the doctors came back in together and spoke with us in low tones.

"It's time to talk about withdrawing care," one of them solemnly told us. "We've done everything we could do, and it's getting to the point that we have to consider if what we are doing is causing more harm than good."

Jennifer had asked me, mere moments before this, if it seemed like we were torturing Larry to keep him here. I posed that question to the doctors. They affirmed that yes, it had pretty much come to that. They suggested we think about removing the ventilator and stopping the infusions of fluids and medications. We discussed this briefly and they graciously gave us some last quiet moments to be alone with Larry.

I held his hand and struggled not to cry as I told this dear man that while I had no wish to see him go, I would try to understand if that's what had to happen. I reminded him that together we had beaten the odds many times and that our faith in God had brought us a long way, but that now it looked like God had another plan in mind. I told him it would be OK, and I loved him. Then it was Jennifer's turn. She stepped forward and took hold of her daddy's hand. She leaned down and told him she loved him, too.

"You've been a good dad, and a good Papa; now it's time for you to go be a good angel, and watch over us from Heaven. It's OK to go, Dad. We'll be OK here."

Within 60 seconds, Larry's heart rate began to drop steadily. Another 60 seconds, and he was gone. He'd taken the agony of turning off those machines out of our hands, and simply left. BJ had been right. Larry just needed his daughter's permission to go home to God.

It was just before 4 am, October 26, 2011.

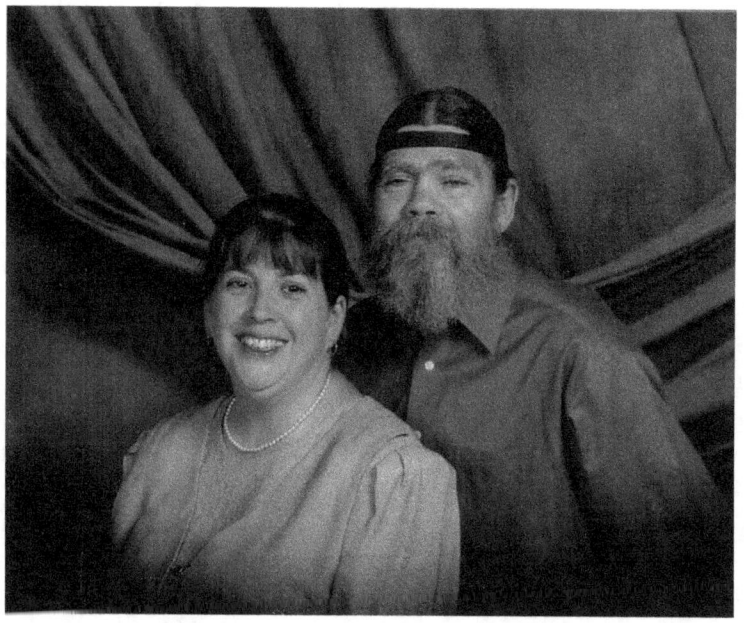

20
HEALING

If you, the reader, have lost someone extremely close to you already, you don't need me to tell you just how shell-shocked we felt; you know only too well. If you haven't, well, I can't recommend it. But it happens to each of us sooner or later, and we all must find our own way through the grief that follows. Faith helps. Friends do what they can to help. But as my mother says (and Mother's always right!), it's a process and there are no shortcuts. So we just keep taking that next step, doing the next thing, even if the "next thing" is just sitting in someone else's favorite comfy chair in a darkened room and wallowing for a while. Just make sure your rear end doesn't grow roots there.

Jennifer and I returned to the hotel to freshen up. She talked to BJ by phone, and they agreed to wait until after school that day to tell the children, when they would all be there together. Knowing my parents probably hadn't slept much overnight, I called them next. Hearing Mother's audible sob was difficult; I would rather take a beating than cause my mother to cry. They had developed a very close relationship with Larry over the years and would mourn his loss greatly. Next came the calls to my sister and brother, to Susan and to Tom, and finally to Larry's dad. I dreaded having to tell Burl, feeling that I had somehow let him down. No parent should have to bury their child, although so many have done just that.

After driving back to the farm, we went into Windsor to make funeral arrangements. We chose flowers, talked with my pastor, and met with the funeral director. Back at the house Jennifer and I went through boxes of family photos, and she spent the next day or more creating a slideshow to play during the visitation, memories of happy times to help us smile. I was careful to get her back home before the school bus arrived that afternoon.

Lily, Luke, Megan, and Ami were devastated by the loss of their Papa. Amid the tears, I talked with each of them by phone after their parents had broken the news, and we struggled to comfort one another. Lily and Luke could recall when Papa was still fairly mobile and able to play. They had formed a very close bond with him in the years when he was their babysitter while Jennifer finished her education. Megan was crushed by Papa's death, but also worried about Grandma having to live alone, and promptly volunteered to come stay with me. (Her parents vetoed the idea, but I thanked her for the offer anyway.) Amarillo, not yet 4 years old, had another concern. Her parents had explained that now Papa lived in Heaven and was healthy and strong and could hear perfectly and had his own teeth and two good legs and, most incredibly, was not in pain anymore and would never be in pain again! This was a lot for her young mind to absorb, and she somehow focused on the prosthetic leg part of all this.

"But what will happen to Papa's stick leg?" she asked.

Her parents didn't know the answer, and let her pose it to me when we spoke on the phone.

"Well, sweetie, that stick leg won't be wasted. I will pack up that leg and the other one we kept in the closet for a spare in case this one broke, and all the special socks that go with them, and take them to the shop where they made that leg for Papa. And those folks will send all that stuff to another country where there aren't as many of those shops and where many of the people are poor and can't buy an artificial leg but someone there will really *need* one. And those stick legs that Papa used will be worked over to fit other people so they can walk around like Papa did, and it will help them," I explained.

"Oh, that will be good," Ami told me, "'cause Papa liked to share!"

* * *

After the funeral, when my sister and her family were about to get in the car to drive back to Texas, Janice mentioned this book. She knew I'd begun the writing while Larry was in the hospital; I think there were only 15 to 20 pages at that point.

"I don't think I can finish it now," I told her. "Who would want to read a book where the hero dies?"

Janice's response caught me a little by surprise: "Well, think about it! Didn't we all read about Anne Frank? Don't you still watch the video of *Steel Magnolias*? And John Wayne in *The Cowboys* and *The Shootist*? The hero doesn't always live, you know. It's *how* they lived that makes them heroic. And Larry did live that way. He was a kind person and a really good listener, and he cared about people and was protective and he had such a calm strength. He wanted to help people, and the purpose of your book is to do that, isn't it? To help people?"

She had a very good point. That was the intended purpose.

"But it will be missing the last part," I told her, "that would've discussed how the transplant helped him and what to expect afterward. Maybe I could talk to some other people who've gotten transplants and include a synopsis of their experiences. I don't want to scare potential recipients into thinking Larry's outcome is typical, because it wasn't."

We agreed to give it some thought and discuss it again later. "If nothing else," Janice told me, "it will be a nice keepsake for the grandkids, to help them know more about Larry when they get older."

She knew that alone would make it worth the effort to me.

* * *

As I write this chapter, the calendar approaches 1 year from the date of Larry's kidney transplant. To say it has been a difficult year would be an oversimplification, but finding words to adequately describe it is a challenge. To have been given the hope that the gift of that kidney brought, only to have that hope crushed so soon afterward was brutal. My immediate question to God was: "Why did you give him such a great kidney if he wasn't going to get to stay here and use it?" The question was followed almost as quickly by what felt to me like God's answer: "Because you'd have always wondered... *what if* he could've just gotten that kidney."

Even so, I struggled with the idea that we had "wasted" a very viable organ. If it had gone to someone else, maybe they wouldn't have died so soon afterward and the gifted kidney could have meant longer life, better health, and more opportunities for that person, as we had hoped it would for Larry. When we'd initially

157

left the hospital, the nurse coordinator had supplied me with a folder that included guidelines for writing a "thank you" note to the donor family, which I had fully intended to do. Now what? What could I possibly write to express my gratitude for the opportunity they'd allowed us? That family was grieving, too; would my message help them or hurt them? Not knowing what to do, I did nothing, but continued to pray that God would heal their hurts.

As for Larry, I believe that he is healed. My faith that he is in Heaven has brought me through this year, and I continue to lean on that belief that Larry is well now, and whole and happy to be in the presence of the Lord, and that when it's my turn to go, I'll see him there.

And if, by chance, God needs warriors, well... he sure got one in Larry.

* * *

I still believe in the transplant process. My driver's license is marked to indicate my willingness to be a donor if the situation presents itself, and my family members have been informed of my wishes. It's sort of the ultimate form of recycling, isn't it? I have read about experimental processes in which new organs are being grown in laboratories and about developments that might eliminate the need for the immune-suppressant drugs that help prevent rejection but can also weaken the patient's system and—as in Larry's case—can mask the symptoms of a brewing infection. Those and other new techniques will likely revolutionize the entire transplant concept before long, and I look forward to hearing about those advances as they come about.

But in the meantime, here are some statistics:

- According to a pamphlet from University Hospital in Columbia, Missouri, as of January 2008, their 1-year success rate for adults with kidney transplants is 93%.

- In their patients who received kidneys from living donors, the success rate at the 1-year mark is 100%, and for patients receiving a kidney from a deceased donor, 92%.

158

- A chart from the U.S. Organ Procurement and Transplantation Network (OPTN) shows that the success rate nationwide for a deceased-donor kidney is 94.5% at 1 year and 81% at 5 years. The rates are better from a living-donor kidney: 97.6% and 89.8%, respectively.

- A transplanted functioning kidney is about five times more effective in replacing overall kidney function than dialysis, which can help the patient feel much better.

- A successful kidney transplant can result in a longer life for the patient than that patient might have if he/she remained on dialysis. One doctor told me that 5 to 10 years is the average life expectancy for a new dialysis patient, as opposed to a 10- to 20-year life expectancy for someone with a transplanted kidney. These are broad ranges, however, and represent a verbal opinion, not documented statistics.

- Generally speaking, wait time for a kidney match on "The List" is longer in the eastern United States than it is in the Midwest. At one point I heard 5 years was the average wait time in the Northeast, compared with 2 years here in Missouri.

* * *

The most common gram-negative organism causing bloodstream infections like the one Larry had is *E. coli*, but there are others. One study I found indicated that this type of infection results in death within 28 days of transplant in only 1.6% of kidney transplant recipients.[i]

I make reference to this to clarify that Larry's death was not a typical result. It is not my wish to discourage anyone from seeking a transplant. However, because I am not able to provide a first-hand account of what might be expected after most kidney transplant surgeries, I've interviewed several people who can. They were all very kind and open in telling me their stories; the following chapter gives a brief summary of their experiences.

159

[i]Incidence Rate and Outcome of Gram-Negative Bloodstream Infection in Solid Organ Recipients by M. N. Al-Hasan, R. R. Razonable, J. E. Eckel-Passow, and L. M. Baddour, published in American Journal of Transplantation, 2009.

http://xa.yimg.com/kq/groups/16781130/254656925/name/bactere mia.pdf

21
THE INTERVIEWS

Larry Fosnow had no idea his kidneys were failing. A busy guy, he and his wife Mary Ann are almost constantly "on the go." Married to each other for more than 40 years, they've raised four children and really enjoy being grandparents. But several years back, Larry was feeling draggy. He'd go to work, tend the yard, try to keep up with all the projects he had going, but just felt like he had no energy. He started getting short of breath after what seemed like the slightest exertion. Tests showed he had restricted blood flow to his heart, and a cardiologist put three stents in his coronary arteries to open them up.

Another problem was discovered during the blood work that accompanied this procedure: Larry's kidneys were failing. At that time they were working at only 18% of full function, leaving a lot of toxins unfiltered from his bloodstream. No wonder he felt so sluggish! A discussion of his history revealed Mr. Fosnow had served his country in the U.S. Army and was wounded in Vietnam. A physical examination at the time of his military discharge had shown some loss of kidney function, and Larry recalled that they kept him in the hospital for about a week before sending him home. No advice was offered at the time regarding dietary restrictions or having his kidneys checked occasionally. At least one doctor has since told him that his exposure in Vietnam to the chemical "Agent Orange" may have contributed to his kidney failure.

Larry was put on the waiting list for a kidney. He received three of the "yellow-alert" calls telling him the team in Kansas City (about 80 miles away) might have an organ for him. He even went to the hospital once, but each time was sent back home to wait some more.

The Fosnows, of course, had talked to their children—now all adults—and told them about the diagnosis. Each of the kids offered to be tested as a possible donor for their dad, and the first to be tested was Lori, who was 30 at the time. Her lab tests confirmed she would be a good match. The surgery was scheduled, and they arrived at the hospital about 6 am, mere hours before the procedure.

After the operation, Larry was kept in the ICU for a day, where they kept a close watch on his heart. No problems ensued, and he was released from the hospital after 5 days. He came home with several prescription drugs, including Cellcept (mycophenolate mofetil), Rapamune (sirolimus), and prednisone. At some point later, Prograf (tacrolimus) was substituted for one of the others. The dosages of his medications are still adjusted by his doctor from time to time, based on the results of blood tests done every 2 months.

At the time of our interview, more than 12 years after his transplant, Larry feels good and he enjoys his busy life. "They made me stay off work 2 or 3 months" after the transplant surgery, he says, although he felt he could have returned sooner. If having his arteries opened up with the stents helped restore some of that lost energy, getting a healthy, working kidney really put him back on track! He doesn't get tired nearly as easily as he did before the transplant, but he is careful about lifting or carrying things. Because a transplanted kidney is typically placed just inside the abdomen, rather than farther back within the body, where our original kidneys are situated, it is not as naturally protected, and he is conscious of this. The other limitation he mentioned: "I can't run a jackhammer." (!)

Larry's advice to anyone with compromised kidneys: "It's really important to watch what you eat." He speculates that his kidneys might have lasted longer if he had been aware of their compromised state and restricted his intake of meat and other proteins.

Larry Fosnow is extremely grateful for the support of his family and for his daughter's gift of a kidney. They were told that anyone who donates a kidney and later loses the function of their remaining kidney is automatically placed at the top of the waiting list to receive a transplant themselves. This news helped to reassure Lori and the rest of the family.

162

*　*　*

In September 2012, I spoke with Carolyn Matthews about her transplant experience.

With a medical history that included diabetes, sleep apnea, and high blood pressure that proved very difficult to control, she was under the care of specialists in nephrology and endocrinology. When she was about 55 years old, she began in-center dialysis, and was on dialysis for more than 2 years before getting a kidney transplant.

Carolyn had two yellow-alert calls before the one preceding her actual surgery took place. When the Big Day finally arrived, she was in the hospital only 4 to 5 hours before the surgery commenced. Five days later, when the central line was removed from the vein in her neck, Carolyn suffered a stroke, probably as a result of a clot that had formed in the area. This setback resulted in another month's stay in the hospital, after which Carolyn stayed with her grown daughter for 6 months while she continued to recuperate.

At the time of our visit, it had been almost 3 years since her transplant. Carolyn sees her doctor quarterly, and he still makes small changes to her medications now and then. "I feel good," she told me. "No more dialysis. I don't get worn out as quickly on outings now. I can go to the Mall and walk around now, and my legs don't feel heavy anymore. I have more energy. I can play with my granddaughter!"

For the first year after her transplant, Carolyn avoided people with colds, and she has not been sick. Her advice to other patients who are hoping for a kidney transplant: "Be patient. Don't skip your dialysis treatments. It will be well worth it!"

*　*　*

Another gentleman we'll call "RG" (at his request) was diagnosed with high blood pressure and high cholesterol in 1996. In 2000, as a result of routine blood tests to monitor these issues, his doctor noticed a rise in RG's creatinine; it had crept from 0.9 to 1.5, and by the next year it was 2.0. On January 1, 2002, at the age of 62, RG celebrated the New Year with a new marriage. The newlyweds waited until June to take a vacation, and it was while they were traveling that RG realized he just didn't feel well. Upon their return home he went to his doctor for a physical, and as a result was referred to a nephrologist, where blood tests determined his kidneys were failing.

Fistula surgery was performed in October 2002, and in January 2003, RG began dialysis treatments. After 7 weeks of in-center dialysis, however, his creatinine dropped back below 3.0, and according to medical guidelines, he was able to discontinue the treatments. His doctor explained that this sometimes happened. While his kidneys weren't "healed," the dialysis had helped enough to win him a hiatus. No one could predict how long this might last; it could be days, weeks, or maybe months.

In this case, the break lasted until February 2004 and helped to alleviate the deep depression that undergoing dialysis had caused him. When his dialysis resumed, RG made the decision to seek a kidney transplant. In July 2004 he began testing in Kansas City, Missouri, and was placed on the transplant waiting list in the fall of that year. Somewhere along the line, it was discovered that RG had only one kidney that was even partially functioning: the other had shriveled to about the size of an English walnut, and doctors couldn't tell him if it had ever worked!

After two of the typical yellow-alert calls, RG received a kidney transplant on February 24, 2007. He'd been called in the early afternoon, was told to be at the hospital by midnight, and had surgery about noon the next day. After the transplant, he was in a private room, and his hospital stay lasted 7 or 8 days. Like many transplant patients, he was sent home with two different medications to prevent organ rejection. After about 4 weeks one of these was reduced, which relieved the side effects of nausea and vomiting RG had been experiencing.

About 3 months after the transplant, RG developed diabetes, but he doesn't know if there is any correlation between the events. His medications have been stabilized now for some time, and he is doing well. Lab reports from the summer of 2012 showed his creatinine levels were between 0.9 and 1.1.

"I enjoy things more now, and have a better appreciation for things," he told me. "I'm more apt to work in the yard, and I've been collecting classic toy tractors. With my son, I started participating in tractor pulls this year." Because the weights that are added to the tractor with each new round of competition weigh 45 pounds or more, RG doesn't change them himself, minding his doctor's restriction. He was also cautioned against eating shrimp or drinking orange and grapefruit juice, and was advised to avoid the jerky motions involved in riding roller coasters, working with horses, or using water skis, so as not to jar the transplanted kidney he received.

Even with having to take immune suppressant medications for the rest of his life—and the expenses associated with that regimen—RG is convinced the benefits of a kidney transplant outweigh the drawbacks. As he told me: "I was handed a second chance; what I do with it is up to me."

* * *

Born and raised in the great state of Texas, Melanie Holmes began the medical journey toward a kidney transplant in 1986, when she was diagnosed with lupus soon after the birth of her first child. Systemic lupus erythematosus (SLE) is an autoimmune disease that affects approximately 3 out of every 10,000 people. Of those affected, 10% to 30% will eventually experience kidney failure as the tiny blood vessels in their kidneys burst and create scar tissue. Melanie received regular medical care from specialists in nephrology and rheumatology. She took several medications to help control the symptoms of high blood pressure, painful joints, and edema (swelling).

"When the doctor first told me I would eventually need a kidney transplant, it made me mad!" Melanie said to me during our telephone interview. "I knew that I was doing everything I had been advised to do to take care of myself, and that I was being as proactive as possible to protect my health." Finally, the doctor explained that it wasn't something she could control. Autoimmune diseases cause the body's immune system to mistake healthy cells and tissue for harmful ones, and then to attack them. Based on her test results, her doctor could see what was happening and just wanted to prepare her for what seemed to him an inevitable result.

By 2005, the time had arrived; Melanie's kidneys were failing. The doctor talked with her about starting dialysis, but several people she knew had volunteered to be tested as potential donors, and the transplant center in Dallas was proceeding with testing the first of those, so they made the decision to put off the treatments a little longer. The news soon afterward that Greg, Melanie's brother-in-law, was an acceptable match, was indeed an answer to prayer.

Melanie and her family live in a suburb of Dallas, so the trip to the hospital took about 50 minutes with the busy traffic in the area. They arrived just a few hours before the prescheduled surgery began, and everything went well. After 1 day in ICU, Melanie was moved to a private room in the hospital. No visitors were allowed because of her weakened immune system. She recalls having a bad reaction to one of the antirejection drugs because it included rabbit serum in its ingredients. "I never knew I was allergic to rabbits before that," she told me. That medication was quickly changed to another, and Melanie returned home after just over a week in the hospital. The big box of medications and the schedule for when to take each one was a bit overwhelming at first. Something in the mix made her hands shake, a symptom she had not previously experienced. Over the course of the next year, however, with her doctor's gradual adjustments to the medications and their dosages, that side effect disappeared. Melanie still takes two drugs (Prograf and Myfortic [mycophenolic acid]) to prevent rejection of the transplanted kidney and does not expect that to change in the future. She also takes medication to control the lupus symptoms, and remains vigilant to prevent any complications that she can. After her kidney transplant, she was able to have several small areas of skin cancer—caused by the lupus—successfully treated. They have now healed well.

I asked Melanie how she feels these days. "Very fortunate!" she told me. "My stamina is so much improved, and my clarity of thinking. The brain fog I was experiencing before is gone. I can stay awake all day now. I feel like I'm *me* again!"

166

As recommended by her doctors, she avoids rare steaks and raw meat like sushi, and protects her skin from overexposure to sunlight. But the benefits far outweigh the drawbacks as far as she's concerned.

When asked for her advice to anyone else who might be facing this type of challenge, Melanie made what seemed to me some very important points:

"Chronic illness and depression often go hand-in-hand. You shouldn't have to feel guilty for feeling bad. There are medications that can help, and it's OK to use those! Don't be afraid. Ask your doctor questions. Educate yourself about your specific condition and the options available to you, and then make the best choice you can and move forward."

* * *

I spoke with Bill and Kay Buck by telephone in September 2012. Bill suffered from polycystic kidney disease (PKD), a hereditary disorder affecting almost 1 in 1,000 Americans. It had caused the death of his brother at age 38. Bill's mother had had PKD as well, and had undergone in-center dialysis before her death from the disease. Bill was diagnosed with PKD at the age of 32, and started taking medication to control the resulting high blood pressure. He also began a special diet in which red meat and salt, among other things, were restricted to help keep his blood pressure under control as much as possible. PKD causes cysts to form in the kidneys, sometimes in clusters. Currently there is no treatment available to prevent or cure this disease. Sometimes the cysts rupture, causing extreme pain. By the time Bill was 52, his kidneys were wearing out, and he began home hemodialysis treatments. He felt very tired, but continued to work at his job. He and his wife Kay researched the available options for transplant, and registered with the program run by Barnes-Jewish Hospital in St Louis, Missouri, about a 2-hour drive from their home.

Kay Buck volunteered to donate a kidney for her husband, and after she passed the tests, a surgery date was set. They checked into the hospital on a Monday evening; the transplant took place on Tuesday morning, July 21, 2009; and they were both back home on Friday of that week! According to Bill: "I felt better following the transplant than I had felt in 20 to 25 years." Food tasted better, the color of his skin and the whites of his eyes had a healthier tone, and he relished the freedom of not being tethered to the dialysis machine. "It's been a true blessing," he told me.

Six medications were prescribed immediately after the transplant, including Prograf, Myfortic, a steroid, low-dose aspirin, and something for high cholesterol. Initially Bill went for blood tests once a week for monitoring. He estimates it took about 3 months of gradual adjustments to the medications before things were somewhat stabilized. Things went along well for the next couple of years, but then monthly blood tests from January and February of 2012 showed elevated levels of blood urea nitrogen (BUN) and creatinine, signs that the transplanted kidney was not functioning as well. By March he was suffering nausea and lack of appetite. Immediately after the lab results from March were done, Bill received a call at work from the transplant department, telling him the doctor wanted to see him at the hospital within 3 hours. Further testing showed he was experiencing a flare-up of the BK virus. He had never heard of it before. Nor had I, until our conversation.

The BK virus was discovered in 1971, when researchers isolated the virus in the urine of a transplant patient with the initials "B.K." First-time BK virus infections occur during early childhood in most people and typically don't produce any symptoms, so nearly everyone who has had BK virus is unaware of it. In reading about this virus, I've learned that about 75% of the human race is likely to test positive for BK virus in their systems, where it can remain dormant for years; it almost never causes symptoms unless or until a person experiences a compromised immune system. Obviously, transplant patients are included in this category because of the immune suppressant drugs that help prevent rejection of the organ they received. However, flare-ups of BK virus do not occur in all kidney recipients; the virus causes a progressive kidney transplant injury in about 1% to 10% of kidney transplant patients, but injury doesn't occur until late in the course of the disease, and early detection and treatment can preserve the long-term life of the transplant.

In Bill's case, the BK virus caused an infection that threatened the survival of the kidney his wife had donated. He underwent a needle biopsy of the kidney on March 21, 2012, and was told the viral count was 40,000. His doctor explained they would discontinue the medication Myfortic in order to give his immune system a chance to fight off the virus. Bill stayed on low doses of Prograf and prednisone for anti-rejection.

The next 6 months were a challenge. Bill was told that occurrences of BK virus flare-ups are typically seen in the first 10 months or so after transplant, but in his case, it had been 32 months. Once again, he was going for weekly blood tests, hoping for good news but dreading what he might hear. At one point the viral count was as high as 4 million, and his creatinine level was up to 4.0. A nurse told Bill he was about 2 weeks away from having to go back on dialysis.

Kay put her husband on a strict diet, which Bill willingly followed. She made fruit smoothies for him to drink, putting in blueberries, raspberries, whatever fruits she could find that were high in antioxidants. Bill drank lots of water to help flush toxins from his system. Eventually, the numbers started looking better. The viral count dropped to 200,000, and then finally hovered between 11,000 and 8,500. He kept waiting for this number to read "zero" but was later told that any reading less than 35,000 on this virus is acceptable. Bill's creatinine went back down to 2.3 once, and now stays around 2.5. The virus did create some scar tissue in his kidney, but he has not gone into rejection and is doing much better now.

When asked about drawbacks, Bill mentioned that he now avoids lake swimming. He does not drink alcoholic beverages or smoke cigarettes anymore, and has no desire to do so. He was initially concerned about the medications and possible side effects, but was nevertheless compliant with his doctor's orders.

Both Bill and Kay are enthusiastic in their encouragement of anyone needing to seek a kidney transplant. Looking back, Kay wishes she could have been tested as a possible matching donor before Bill had to begin dialysis, thinking that maybe they could have pre-empted that step. No one mentioned the possibility to them beforehand, but later in the process a nurse told them it might have been feasible. All things considered, however, they are glad for their present outcome. "You have to be your own best advocate. The quality of life after a kidney transplant is well worth it," they agreed.

FURTHER INFORMATION

For readers who want to know more, here are some sources for more information about diabetes and kidney transplantation:

National Kidney Foundation
Online at www.kidney.org
Or by phone:
1-800-622-9010
212-889-2210
Or by mail:
National Kidney Foundation
30 East 33rd Street
New York, NY 10016
****

UNOS (United Network for Organ Sharing)
Online: www.unos.org

Or by mail:
Post Office Box 2484
Richmond, Virginia 23218
****

National Kidney Registry
Online: www.kidneytransplantcenters.org
Or by mail:
National Kidney Registry
P.O. Box 460
Babylon, NY 11702-0460
****

American Diabetes Association
Online: www.diabetes.org
By phone: 1-800-DIABETES (1-800-342-2383)
By mail:
American Diabetes Association
1701 North Beauregard Street
Alexandria, VA 22311

www.ingramcontent.com/pod-product-compliance
Lightning Source LLC
Chambersburg PA
CBHW060509290526
45791CB00001B/336